MINIMAL Access

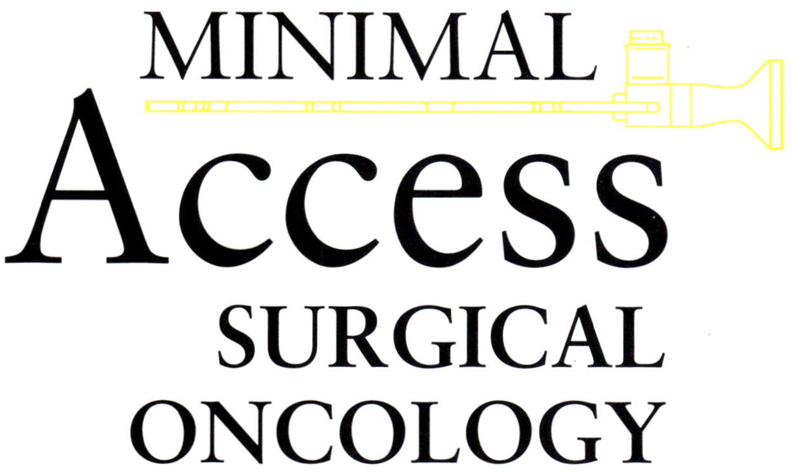

SURGICAL ONCOLOGY

Edited by Frederick L Greene

University of South Carolina School of Medicine,
Columbia, USA

and

R David Rosin

St Mary's Hospital, London, UK

Foreword by Alfred Cuschieri

Ninewells Hospital and Medical School, Dundee, UK

RADCLIFFE MEDICAL PRESS, OXFORD AND NEW YORK

Radcliffe Medical Press Ltd
18 Marcham Road, Abingdon, Oxon OX14 1AA, UK

Radcliffe Medical Press, Inc.
141 Fifth Avenue, New York, NY 10010, USA

British Library Cataloguing in Publication Data

A catalogue record for this book is available from the British Library.

ISBN 1 85775 080 2

Library of Congress Cataloging-in-Publication Data

Minimal access surgical oncology/edited by Frederick L. Greene and
  R. David Rosin: foreword by Alfred Cuschieri.
      p. cm.
    Includes bibliographical references and index.
    ISBN 1-85775-080-2
    1. Cancer—Endoscopic surgery. I. Greene, Frederick L.
  II. Rosin, R. David.
    [DNLM: 1. Neoplasms—surgery.   2. Surgery, Laparoscopic—methods.
  QZ 268 M665 1995]
  RD651.M56 1995
  616.994059—dc20
  DNLM/DLC
  for Library of Congress   95–5161
                                                                  CIP

Contents

List of contributors   v

Foreword   vii

Introduction   ix

1   Philosophy of minimal access surgery   1
ROBERT W BEART JR

2   Diagnostic techniques in abdominal evaluation   4
DAVID W EASTER and NANCY L FURUMOTO

3   Laparoscopic staging of malignancy for the upper   21
gastrointestinal tract and pancreas
FREDERICK L GREENE

4   Laparoscopic staging of abdominal lymphomas   31
ALAN T LEFOR

5   Techniques of abdominal lymph node evaluation,   45
biopsy and dissection
THOMAS A STELLATO

6   Laparoscopic biliary and gastric bypass   57
R DAVID ROSIN and SIMON PATERSON-BROWN

7	Laparoscopic evaluation and resection of the spleen in cancer management EDWARD H PHILLIPS and RAUL J ROSENTHAL	63
8	Laparoscopic resection of the colon and rectum BRUCE V MACFADYEN JR and CHARLES R MATHIS	90
9	Laparoscopic resection of adrenal masses DAVID M ALBALA and RICHARD A PRINZ	109
10	Laparoscopic placement of enteral feeding tubes DAVID M OTA and STEVEN STANDIFORD	119
11	Thoracoscopic evaluation and resection in pulmonary malignancy MICHAEL J MACK, STEPHEN R HAZELRIGG and RODNEY J LANDRENEAU	134
12	Laparoscopic approach for regional hepatic chemotherapy in the treatment of primary or metastatic malignancy MORRIS E FRANKLIN JR, RICHARD F NOREM and RICHARD STUBBS	153
13	Port-site metastasis RAGHU S SAVALGI and R DAVID ROSIN	158
14	Oncological risks in laparoscopic surgery JEAN MOUIEL, FRANCESCO CRAFA, RAFFAELE CURSIO, ROBERT STUBINSKI and JEAN GUGENHEIM	166
15	Future trends in minimal access surgery: telepresence surgery and virtual reality IRWIN B SIMON	183
Index		187

List of contributors

David M Albala, Department of Urology, Loyola University Medical Center, Maywood, Illinois, USA

Robert W Beart, Department of Surgery, University of Southern California, Los Angeles, California, USA

Francesco Crafa, St Roch Hospital, Nice, France

Raffaele Cursio, St Roch Hospital, Nice, France

David W Easter, University of California, San Diego Medical Center, San Diego, California, USA

Morris E Franklin Jr, Southeast Surgical Office, San Antonio, Texas, USA

Nancy L Furumoto, University of California, San Diego Medical Center, San Diego, California, USA

Frederick L Greene, University of South Carolina School of Medicine, Columbia, South Carolina, USA

Jean Gugenheim, St Roch Hospital, Nice, France

Stephen R Hazelrigg, Southern Illinois University, Springfield, Illinois, USA

Rodney L Landreneau, University of Pittsburg, Pittsburg, Pennsylvania, USA

Alan T Lefor, University of Maryland at Baltimore, Baltimore, Maryland, USA

Bruce V Macfadyen Jr, The University of Texas Medical School, Houston, Texas, USA

Michael J Mack, Medical City Dallas Hospital, Dallas, Texas, USA

Charles R Mathis, The University of Texas Medical School, Houston, Texas, USA

Jean Mouiel, St Roch Hospital, Nice, France

Richard F Norem, Alexandria, Louisiana, USA

David M Ota, University of Missouri-Columbia, Ellis Fischel Cancer Center, Columbia, Missouri, USA

Simon Paterson-Brown, Royal Infirmary, Edinburgh, UK

Edward H Phillips, Cedars-Sinai Medical Center, Los Angeles, California, USA

Richard A Prinz, Department of Surgery, Rush University Medical School, Chicago, Illinois, USA

Raul J Rosenthal, Cedars-Sinai Medical Center, Los Angeles, California, USA

R David Rosin, St Mary's Hospital, London, UK

Raghu S Savalgi, Yale University School of Medicine, New Haven, Connecticut, USA

Irwin B Simon, University of Nevada School of Medicine, Las Vegas, Nevada, USA

Steven Standiford, University of Missouri-Columbia, Ellis Fischel Cancer Center, Columbia, Missouri, USA

Thomas A Stellato, Case-Western Reserve University, Ireland Cancer Center, Cleveland, Ohio, USA

Richard Stubbs, Wakefield Surgical Clinic, Newtown, Wellington, New Zealand

Robert Stubinski, St Roch Hospital, Nice, France

Foreword

Perhaps, there are few areas of surgical practice which have caused more anxiety and debate than the minimal surgical approach to malignant intra-abdominal and intra-thoracic disease. The benefits of staging by laparoscopy and, more recently by thoracoscopy, are established and have been enhanced by the advent of contact ultrasonography, performed during these minimal access staging procedures which often obviate unnecessary open intervention in patients with incurable disease. The developments over the past five years, however, have gone beyond this, such that both palliative and potentially curative, ablative operations are now practised via the endoscopic or endoscopically-assisted approach.

There is obviously a watershed at which benefit from the minimal access approach in the management of malignant disorders is either unproved, unlikely to materially benefit the patient or indeed may jeopardize outcome and disease-free survival. An objective, up-to-date account of the present stage of minimal access surgery in the management of intra-abdominal and intra-thoracic malignancies was overdue. This is now provided by *Minimal Access Surgical Oncology* which is comprehensive whilst stressing the areas of concern, such as the risk of tumor dissemination and port-site recurrences, and the need for clinical trials or prospective centralized evaluation before routine adoption of some of the novel minimal access surgical procedures. It will probably take some time, at least another ten years, before the precise role of minimal access surgery is defined in the management of various oncological disorders. Meantime, *Minimal Access Surgical Oncology* has set the scene and the two editors are to be congratulated for recruiting an excellent panel of contributors and for producing a well-balanced, concise account which is high on facts and short on speculation.

Alfred Cuschieri
February 1995

Introduction

No group of patients can benefit more from recent advances in minimal access surgery than those patients with abdominal and thoracic malignancy. Our goal as physicians has always been to tackle cancer in its earliest form, and to intervene when tumors are small and potentially curable by surgical extirpative techniques. In association with more traditional imaging modalities (computed tomography, ultrasonography, nuclear medicine scanning and magnetic resonance imaging), diagnostic laparoscopy can help to confirm a tumor in the abdominal cavity. The goal of both laparoscopy and these traditional imaging techniques is to assist in the appropriate staging of patients who may not in fact be candidates for major surgical resection. Today, when adjuvant radiation and chemotherapy have become so important for many patients who have solid tumors and malignancy of the reticuloendothelial system involving the abdominal cavity, this quest for appropriate staging is of particular relevance.

As the laparoscope and the thoracoscope become routine tools for the diagnosis and staging of abdominal and thoracic tumors, minimal access techniques for resection and bypass will continue to advance. This monograph is devoted to the descriptions of initial diagnosis, staging and therapeutic modalities that can be used on a daily basis for the management of our patients with cancer.

We dedicate this monograph to the thousands of patients who will benefit from the use of minimal access surgical techniques that lead to potential cure and greater comfort. As William Osler said many years ago, 'Diseases that harm call for therapies that harm less.'

Frederick L Greene, MD
R David Rosin, MD
February 1995

Philosophy of minimal access surgery

ROBERT W BEART JR

Minimal access surgery has evolved rapidly since the start of the decade. It is generally acknowledged that this procedure originated in private practice and was largely rejected by academic centers in its early phases. Only after patient demand mandated that this technique be incorporated in all phases of American surgical practice has this procedure been subjected to the scrutiny that a new procedure justly deserves. This raises the question of the philosophy of how new surgical techniques evolve. It is generally conceded that complication rates in one's early experience with laparoscopic cholecystectomy are relatively high and careful evaluation and evolution are necessary if we are to minimize the morbidity of evolving technology. It is the purpose of this chapter to examine the philosophy behind the evolution of this new technology and try to put forward concepts which will guide advances in the future.

Laparoscopic surgery is not used to perform any procedures which have not been previously performed by open techniques. We are trying to do the same procedures in ways that will offer patients the advantage of decreased morbidity while maintaining the traditional standards of cure and palliation.

A new procedure must not compromise the traditional standards offered by the traditional procedure. It must not increase the morbidity and/or mortality, even if it does offer advantages in length of hospital stay or other objective measurements. It seems somewhat schizophrenic that we advertise on the one hand maintaining the traditional surgical standards while on the other hand recognizing that if we are going to take advantage of this new technology, we must change the paradigms of management. Careful examination of these paradigms is necessary to ensure that advantages of adequate surgical treatment are maintained, while at the same time making greatest use of technical advantages offered by new procedures. We should also not change our surgical indications. The fact that we can do a laparoscopic procedure does not lower our indications for surgery or make us more likely to take patients to the operating room. Finally, there are cases that are inappropriate for laparoscopic procedures: cases where the entire abdomen must be carefully inspected, such as in patients with a bowel obstruction or extensive known adhesive disease.

In an effort to maintain traditional standards while at the same time taking advantage of the new technology, we have evolved several principles. First, we maintain a low threshold for abandonment of the procedure. If at any time we feel that a procedure comparable to the open procedure cannot be performed, or if the procedure is going to be unduly prolonged, the procedure will be abandoned. Secondly, adequate exposure must be maintained to provide a margin of safety throughout the procedure. If at any time we run the risk of losing control of blood vessels, we will abandon the procedure. Third, we avoid undue prolongation of the procedure. An alarm clock is placed in the operating room to ring at the moment when the procedure would have been finished had it been done as an open procedure. If the procedure is not well along its way by this time, it is usually abandoned in favor of the open technique. Fourth, we have carefully defined our margins of resection and points of vessel ligation to maintain our traditional emphasis on the wide resection of cancers. If we cannot maintain these values, then the procedure is converted to the open technique. We also feel that quoting conversion rates is counterproductive. There is no such thing as an 'excessive' conversion rate. At the point where the surgeon feels that the patient is not being well served by the technique, then it should be abandoned, regardless of the impact on the surgeon's rate of conversion. These statistics should not be tracked. It should not be considered a complication if the procedure is converted from a laparoscopic procedure to an open procedure.

On the other hand, we can and should take advantage of the new surgical technology by changing our traditional management. It appears that most patients after laparoscopic abdominal surgery retain their bowel function and can eat early. We therefore offer patients a liquid diet as soon as they are alert. As a result, we are able to decrease parenteral pain medication requirements and offer patients an earlier release from hospital and return to work. We have adopted the philosophy of starting all procedures laparoscopically, unless there is a known history of extensive intra-abdominal adhesions (though now recognized that a history of multiple previous abdominal surgery is not in itself an indication that there will be extensive adhesive disease).

Certification for surgeons performing laparoscopy is still evolving. It is important to adopt an institutional philosophy which will safeguard the welfare of the patient, while not being so cumbersome that it inhibits the future evolution and development. There are several principles which seem important. First, if the physician is going to attempt a procedure with minimal access techniques, he should also be credentialed to do it as an open procedure. Secondly, physicians who are initiating new procedures should probably be assisted for a specified number of cases by surgeons who have at least the same level of training and are qualified to do the procedures with the open technique as well. This should help when making judgements during the learning phase. Although clinical and/or educational courses are of great value to physicians, it is unrealistic to expect physicians to attend courses for every procedure which they intend to perform.

Additional philosophical issues relate to technical issues. We feel that videotaping of the procedures is advantageous. Videotapes should not be considered a part of the medical record but as part of the educational process, and it is appropriate to destroy them routinely after a 30-day interval. Keeping them available for 30 days is desirable in case a delayed complication occurs. Lower levels of intra-abdominal pressures are necessary when extensive intra-abdominal resections are carried out. We keep the use of 10 mm ports to a minimum since hernias are prone to occur through them. The two-handed technique is mandatory for extensive intra-abdominal procedures.

New procedures are desirable for our patients. It is important, however, that these procedures evolve in a controlled way that results in careful evaluation as to their safety and efficacy. At the same time, it is also important that the credentialing process is not so cumbersome that we inhibit the evolution of new procedures. A thoughtful philosophy of evolution can achieve both of these goals. We feel the principles we have laid down have guided us in the safe and rapid evolution of this technology in our environment.

2

Diagnostic techniques in abdominal evaluation

DAVID W EASTER and NANCY L FURUMOTO

Introduction

Along with the exponential growth of technology in minimal access surgery, there has been a revival in the use of diagnostic laparoscopy and thoracoscopy in both oncologic and non-oncologic diseases. Diagnostic laparoscopy with biopsy can be utilized in primary diagnosis and staging as well as in second-look procedures. If unresectability is determined upon laparoscopic examination, palliative methods (done either laparoscopically, endoscopically or by other means) can reduce the number and morbidity of open laparotomy cases. Laparoscopic biopsy techniques do not differ significantly from open techniques, but offer an important intermediary position in the continuum of available tissue-sampling methods, ie radiographic-directed biopsy to open surgery.

This chapter discusses the history, indications, contraindications, advantages, disadvantages and possible complications of diagnostic laparoscopy with biopsy for oncologic diseases. Operative techniques are described, and future directions and applications are discussed.

History

The first documented laparoscopic visualization of the peritoneal cavity was in 1901 by the Russian gynecologist Ott[1], who performed a culdotomy and named his procedure 'ventroscopy'. In the same year, Kelling[2] performed celioscopy on dogs by creating a pneumoperitoneum with room air and then inserting a trocar and cystoscope for visual examination of the abdomen. In 1910, Jakobeus[3] was the first to use the term 'laparoscopy' and to describe the use of a cystoscope for examining patients with ascites (for which he did not use a pneumoperitoneum). He described the use of the laparoscope to confirm the diagnosis of cirrhosis, metastatic tumor and tuberculus peritonitis[4]. The first laparoscopy in the USA was performed in 1911 at Johns Hopkins Hospital by Bernheim[5].

At first, visualization was limited by the use of the cystoscope which offered only an acute angle of vision. By the late 1920s, forward-viewing scopes had been developed which increased the viewing angle to 135°. In 1929, Kalk[6] described a dual puncture technique and also pioneered the use of laparoscopy for liver and biliary disease. Fervers[7] in 1933 emphasized the importance of using carbon dioxide or oxygen instead of room air for pneumoperitoneum. He also reported his experience with 50 patients and described therapeutic laparoscopy for the first time (lysis of adhesions). In the 1930s, Ruddock and Benedict were early proponents of laparoscopy with biopsy in North America. In 1934, Ruddock[8] used monopolar cautery with biopsy forceps for the first time. Benedict[9] described the use of laparoscopy in the diagnosis of liver disease, ascites, gynecological diseases, gastric cancer, and colonic neoplasms. In 1938, Verres[10] introduced a spring-loaded needle to instill gas for pneumothorax which later was used for pneumoperitoneum.

A major improvement in the optics for laparoscopy occurred in 1952 when Hopkins[11] devised the glass rod-air lens system. In the 1970s, further refinements in instrumentation and techniques centered in Germany[12]. In the 1980s and 1990s improvements in fiberoptics to increase light transmission and the coupling of the laparoscope to a micro-chip camera and video monitor have produced a clear image that assistants can view simultaneously. Technical advances in both instrumentation and visualization are currently occurring almost daily. Although the use of diagnostic laparoscopy for malignant diseases dates back to Jakobeus in 1910, the many refinements over the last 80 years have revived the utility of this approach for the diagnosis and accurate staging of malignant diseases.

Indications

Laparoscopic-directed tissue biopsy should be considered whenever other less invasive methods fail to identify the cause of symptoms. This decision is based on both sound clinical judgement and the level of expertise in laparoscopic-directed biopsy and diagnosis in one's community. Laparoscopic biopsy can be seen as an intermediate level of invasiveness between radiographic-directed biopsy and open laparotomy. A recent case report illustrates the ability of this approach[13].

A 16-year-old female was diagnosed with Ewing's sarcoma involving the left pelvis, and she was treated with chemotherapy. Seven months after diagnosis, however, she was readmitted with fever, neutropenia and upper respiratory infection symptoms. She subsequently developed jaundice, elevated liver function and thrombocytopenia, and computed tomography (CT) revealed multiple hepatic and splenic lesions. A radiographic-directed percutaneous liver aspirate did not demonstrate malignant cells. A week later, another liver aspirate was done with radiographic-directed guidance, revealing a few cells consistent with malignancy, but the sample was insufficient for histochemical and immunologic studies to confirm the diagnosis. A laparoscopic-directed core needle biopsy of the right lobe of the liver was done next, and metastatic Ewing's sarcoma to the liver was confirmed. Although the patient was high-risk for bleeding due to thrombocytopenia with liver function abnormalities, the laparoscopic-directed biopsy was successful in that:

- tissue for diagnosis was obtained safely

- the extent of disease was surveyed

- hemostasis was provided instantly after biopsy

- an unnecessary open laparotomy was avoided

- guidance was obtained about the future care of this patient.

Another indication for diagnostic laparoscopy and directed biopsy is for the staging of a patient with known neoplasia. This is often necessary to plan the treatment and care of oncologic patients appropriately. It has been shown to be especially useful in malignancies that frequently metastasize to the liver or peritoneal surfaces (ie pancreatic, esophageal and gastric malignancies). These small-volume metastases are often missed with computed tomography or ultrasonography but are clearly seen with diagnostic laparoscopy.

The value of diagnostic laparoscopy should increase further with new technical applications such as laparoscopic-directed ultrasonography. One could argue that, regardless of the laparoscopic results, an open laparotomy will often be required. However, with the current level of laparoscopic tissue-handling techniques available (particularly suturing), many patients may be candidates for either laparoscopic completion of a therapeutic procedure or for significant changes in their surgical management because of the results of diagnostic laparoscopy[14].

Contraindications

Laparoscopy and tissue biopsy are contraindicated in only a few situations (Table 2.1). It is obviously *not* indicated when the results of the test will have no valuable response, in other words when the future treatment of the patient will not be affected by the findings of laparoscopy or biopsy. Directed biopsy at laparoscopy is also contraindicated when the risks of the procedure itself are excessive. This is especially important in patients with marginal cardiopulmonary reserve, where the effects of pneumoperitoneum might carry excessive risk.

Relative contraindications to laparoscopy include:

- uncorrectable coagulopathy

- uncontrollable ascites

- limited cardiopulmonary reserve

Absolute	Relative
No possibility of obtaining valuable results	Uncorrectable coagulopathy
Excessive risks (ie severe limited cardiopulmonary reserve)	Uncontrollable ascites
	Limited cardiopulmonary reserve
	Significant abdominal distension from bulky tumors or pregnancy
	Significant adhesions

Table 2.1:   Contraindications to diagnostic laparoscopy.

- significant abdominal distension from large bulky tumors or pregnancy

- significant intraperitoneal adhesions.

In reality, however, many of the relative contraindications to laparoscopy are also the reason why carefully directed laparoscopic biopsy with visual control and hemostasis of the biopsy site is the preferred method of obtaining tissue. With preoperative control of a coagulopathy or ascites, or with careful hemodynamic monitoring with a pulmonary artery catheter in patients with limited cardiopulmonary reserve, laparoscopy can offer a safe method of obtaining tissue in these high-risk patients.

The surgeon should also be aware at all times of the limitations inherent in laparoscopy, the problems that the individual patient presents (ie dense adhesions, confusing anatomy or difficult control of hemostasis due to coagulopathy), and the level of his/her own expertise. Only by recognizing these real limitations will one know quickly when conversion to open laparotomy is indicated.

Advantages vs disadvantages

One very important advantage to diagnostic laparoscopy and laparoscopic-directed biopsy is the ability to diagnose and stage oncologic diseases and to supplement information gained from less invasive tests. With this added information, surgical decision-making is enhanced, and the best next step in treatment (whether for cure or palliation) can be taken. In some cases, open laparotomy can be avoided and palliative measures performed laparoscopically, endoscopically or by other minimal access means.

This approach has been used in a prospective study of 88 consecutive patients with pancreatic or ampullary cancer, comparing the diagnostic accuracy of contrast-enhanced CT, magnetic resonance imaging, angiography and laparoscopy[15]. Laparoscopy with biopsy detected 22 of 23 instances of small liver (less than 2 cm) and peritoneal metastases. Computed tomography detected only two of these small liver metastatic lesions. Fully 89% of unresectable cases could be identified preoperatively using multimodal diagnostic tests, and the combined absence of any positive test result produced a 78% and 100% resectability rate in cancers of the pancreatic head and ampulla, respectively. The study demonstrates the benefit of improved diagnostic accuracy when determining resectability of pancreatic cancer before open surgery attempts at cure or palliation.

In a study of 40 patients with pancreatic adenocarcinoma but in whom no metastases were demonstrable by ultrasound or CT, 17 of 40 patients had undetected metastatic lesions as assessed by preoperative tests. Laparoscopy revealed 14 of 17 patients with metastases[16], necessitating a change in the operative plan.

In another study of 120 patients with undiagnosed abdominal symptoms and/or suspected cancer, diagnostic laparoscopy was 100% accurate in the diagnosis or exclusion of intra-abdominal malignant neoplasms; and subsequent treatment was routinely affected by this information[14]. In 90 patients, laparoscopy was more sensitive and more accurate than ultrasound and/or computed tomography for detecting liver, nodal and peritoneal metastases.

Another advantage of laparoscopic-directed biopsy is seen in patients who are at high risk for operation (ie those with coagulopathy, ascites, immunosuppression or limited cardiopulmonary reserve), yet who would benefit from a tissue diagnosis by a less invasive method than open laparotomy. For example, a patient with acquired immune deficiency syndrome (AIDS) had elevated liver enzymes, right upper quadrant pain, a palpable liver and spleen, and ascites[17]. A CT scan showed no intrahepatic lesions, and a liver/spleen scan showed hepatomegaly but no focal defects. Laparoscopy revealed multiple 2–3 mm purplish nodules on the surface of the liver. Deep-core needle biopsies and superficial punch biopsies of both lobes were obtained, confirming a diagnosis of Kaposi's sarcoma of the liver. The diagnosis was obtained with minimal risk to the patient, and the authors also suggested that less exposure of the operating team to body fluids was possible with the laparoscopic technique.

The advantages of laparoscopic-directed biopsy were also seen in a prospective study of 100 patients with previously undiagnosed liver disease; it enabled a definitive diagnosis to be made in 21 of the patients. Eleven patients had false-negative ultrasound-directed or percutaneous liver biopsies and four patients had peritoneal carcinomatosis where laparoscopy was the only test to suggest unresectable disease.

There are, of course, significant limitations to diagnostic laparoscopy, particularly the loss of the sense of touch. Although not yet fully evaluated, the application of ultrasound- Doppler- and/or radioimmunologic-guided probes may partially compensate for the lack of tactile sensation. Another problem inherent to laparoscopy arises when blood or debris obscures the visual field. Hemostasis and careful dissection are essential for safe laparoscopic surgery.

The complications of laparoscopy (ie trocar injury, effects of pneumoperitoneum, air embolus), are in addition to the risks of tissue biopsy. Finally, exposure of the intended biopsy site can be difficult with laparoscopic methods. Optimal positioning of the patient and proper placement of the operating ports can minimize this limitation.

Techniques

The range of options available for tissue sampling during laparoscopy is equivalent to those with open surgery, with one exception: large specimens require special removal techniques. Two types of samples can be obtained laparoscopically: samples for cytology or tissue for histology. Samples for cytology can be in the form of peritoneal washings, aspiration of fluid or ascites, scrapings, fine needle aspiration or touch preparations. Samples for histology can be in the form of incisional or excisional biopsies. Incisional biopsy techniques include shave, pinch, core and wedge biopsies. If the lesion is exophytic, then shave or pinch biopsy techniques are used. If the lesion is endophytic or deep in the substance of a solid organ, then core or wedge biopsy techniques are used. Excisional techniques are used mainly for lymph node biopsies, where the removal of the intact node is important for accurate pathologic interpretation. Retraction, exposure and mobilization for appropriate biopsy can be problematic during laparoscopic surgery, but there is no organ of the peritoneal or retroperitoneal spaces that is excluded from laparoscopic access techniques.

When the size of the specimen exceeds 1 cm in diameter, common laparoscopic cannulae cannot be used for tissue extraction without morcellation. Options for tissue removal include liquefaction, blunt morcellation (Figure 2.1), increasing cannula size (up to 35 mm as currently available), and simple enlargement of an incision to accommodate the specimen. Our preference is to be quick to enlarge an incision and thereby avoid the other costly and cumbersome alternatives. This approach serves to minimize the cost and complexity of surgery, as well as to provide tissue for pathologic study in as pristine condition as possible.

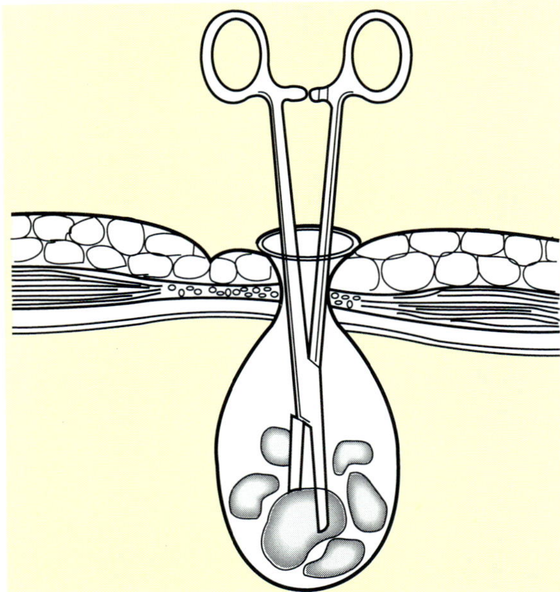

Figure 2.1: Large tissue specimens can be withdrawn in a collection bag after breaking the specimen into smaller pieces. This can be accomplished either with tissue forceps or with finger disruption.

In certain situations, the visual inspection alone during laparoscopy is more informative than biopsy specimens. This is particularly true for peritoneal tuberculosis, where the diagnostic picture is quite accurate and can certainly be obtained much more quickly than if pathologic or microbiologic confirmation is required. Treatment decisions can be made on the visual appearance of tuberculosis with about 95% accuracy[19]. When malignancy is present, the visual diagnosis of carcinomatosis is usually not subtle. Biopsy confirmation is always recommended in these situations, but the visual staging of disease is the most useful information altering both the patient's initial treatment and the ultimate prognosis.

Cytologic sampling at laparoscopy

Cells for cytologic examination can be collected in a number of ways, including peritoneal washings, aspiration of fluid, scrape specimens, fine needle aspiration and touch preparations. A real value of these methods is the potential for rapid diagnosis at the time of sampling. When done in coordination with the surgical pathologist, results from cytology specimens can be as quick and accurate as those from frozen section specimens. The limitations and preferences of one's surgical pathologist/cytologist must be considered prior to sampling, as well as the requirements for tissue architecture, such as with touch preparations for the diagnosis of lymphoma.

For most situations, the aspiration of ascites for diagnosis is best done without the assistance of diagnostic laparoscopy. Patients with a severe coagulopathy may be an exception; however, diagnostic laparoscopy is probably the most sensitive imaging tool to reveal ascites, and if found in association with suspected carcinoma, positive cytology results mean that resection for cure is impossible. During the course of diagnostic laparoscopy, directed lavage and cytologic sampling can reveal otherwise unsuspected peritoneal metastases[20].

Aspiration of peritoneal fluid is easily performed with visual laparoscopic guidance using either a 3 or 5 mm laparoscope. A long narrow gauge needle (as used for central vein catheterizations) is used to pierce the abdominal wall to aspirate fluid collections in any part of the abdomen. Culdocentesis is another access route that can be utilized via the posterior vaginal fornix. Alternatively, an accessory 5 mm cannula may be placed for tissue manipulation and aspiration with laparoscopic instrumentation (Figure 2.2).

Except for the aspiration of ascites, the collection of cytology specimens is best done through a small laparoscopic cannula. This not only permits multiple instrument passes without additional trauma to the abdominal wall, but also limits the contact of neoplastic or infected tissue or fluid to the abdominal wall. Although there are no controlled studies addressing this issue, tumor implantation at the site of laparoscopic manipulation or accessory trocar sites is a well known complication, and one should take every precaution to prevent it.

Fine needle aspiration from solid organs can be easily accomplished under laparoscopic guidance using similar techniques. The advantage of laparoscopic-directed aspiration is the direct visualization of biopsied organs which ensures complete hemostasis by the application of direct pressure, cautery or

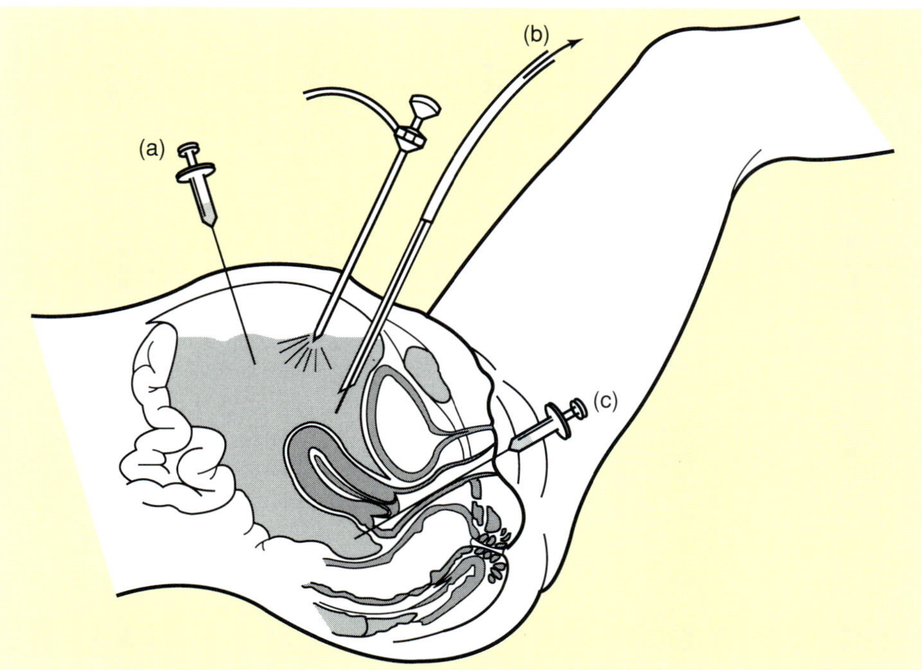

Figure 2.2:   The three common routes of access for fluid aspiration at laparoscopic surgery include: (**a**) direct puncture with a long needle through the abdominal wall, (**b**) aspiration through a laparoscopic cannula, (**c**) aspiration, as in culdocentesis, through the posterior vaginal fornix.

topical hemostatic agents. This capability is a particular advantage when sampling highly vascular organs such as the spleen or liver.

Other cytology preparations are easily collected with laparoscopic guidance. Blunt-nosed forceps, spatula or biopsy scoops (Figures 2.3 and 2.4) can be used for this purpose.

Histologic sampling at laparoscopy

Samples for histologic examination include either incisional or excisional biopsies. Incisional biopsy techniques include shave, pinch, wedge or core needle biopsies. The biopsy method chosen should be the same as if the procedure was done during open surgery. For example if core biopsy is preferable (such as with cirrhosis of the liver), the same sampling is accomplished with laparoscopic techniques.

A spring-loaded core biopsy needle is ideal for use in laparoscopic surgery and reproducibly yields good quality specimens with intact architecture. When biopsies are taken of the liver or spleen, forceps capable of delivering electrocautery are positioned 'at the ready' through an accessory cannula while the core needle is placed through the abdominal wall directly above the biopsy site. In a quick and controlled sequence, the biopsy is taken, the needle is removed,

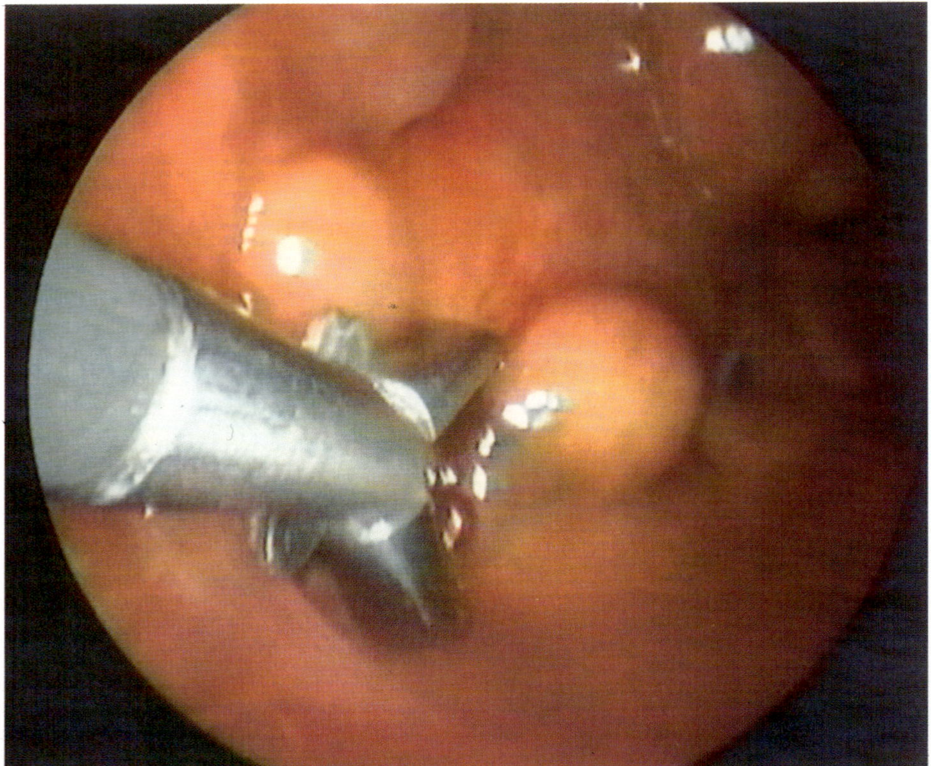

Figure 2.3:   Many laparoscopic instruments are suitable for obtaining scrape specimens for cytology. This operative photograph shows a malignant mesothelioma being sampled with pinching forceps.

and pressure is applied with blunt forceps on the biopsy site. Multiple specimens can be taken in different directions through a single puncture site. After a few minutes of direct pressure on the biopsy site, a short burst of electrocautery is usually sufficient to achieve exact hemostasis. In this way, many areas of concern can be sampled repeatedly, quickly and with complete control of bleeding (Figure 2.5).

Pathologic specimens larger than core samples or cytology preparations require a minimum of three cannulae: one for the laparoscope, one for forceps to hold the tissue, and one for mechanical dissection. Cannulae are best placed after the initial visual inspection of the peritoneal cavity. The angle of dissection should be neither too narrow nor too wide, and should straddle the right and left side of the laparoscope. The angle between instruments and specimen should be between 90° and 135°. This is especially important in more advanced laparoscopic techniques such as suturing.

Shave biopsy specimens can be taken using pinching forceps, scissors or electrocautery dissection. Forceps with teeth are often useful when holding scirrhous carcinomas, but if tissue is too rubbery, firm or friable, a suture can be placed through the intended biopsy site to assist in specimen handling (Figure 2.6). Electrocautery is used sparingly so as to minimize alteration of the pathologic specimen.

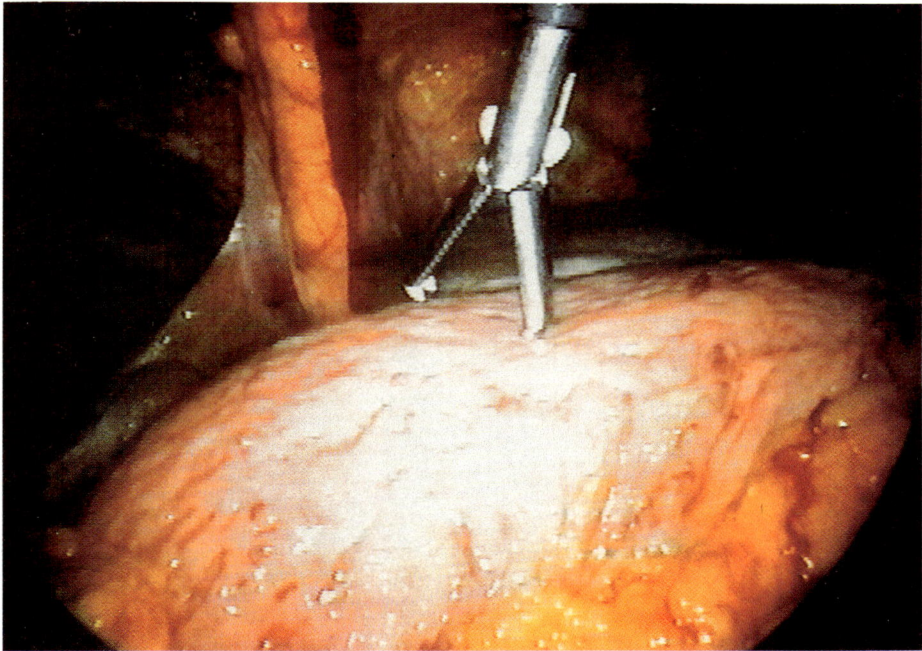

Figure 2.4:   Scrape cytology samples can be taken from firm tissue with the assistance of toothed forceps, as in this case of metastatic breast carcinoma covering the surface of the stomach.

For excisional biopsies, the goal is to remove suspicious tissue in its entirety. Keeping the relationship intact between pathologic and normal tissue facilitates the grading and subtyping of malignancies. Methods of laparoscopic tissue manipulation are similar to those used in open surgery. A collection bag offers potential advantages for specimen handling, in that multiple specimens can be collected for one-step removal and the abdominal wall and other organs are kept shielded from contamination by the specimen. There are many brands of specimen removal bags currently available, each slightly different and offering some potential advantages.

A simple, cost-effective and widely available tissue collection and removal bag is always available as a part of a heavy-duty surgical glove. A finger of the glove is cut at the base, leaving a bowl-shaped opening and a tab on one side that is used for instrument manipulation (Figure 2.7). After tissue dissection, the collection bag is either withdrawn through a large cannula or removed as one commonly removes the gallbladder at laparoscopic surgery. This is done by withdrawing the neck of the bag into the cannula, holding the bag firmly and then withdrawing the instrument/cannula/bag/specimen assembly until the neck of the bag protrudes beyond the abdominal wall. The incision is then either enlarged to accommodate the specimen and bag, or the tissue is removed piecemeal through the mouth of the bag (Figure 2.8).

(a) (b)

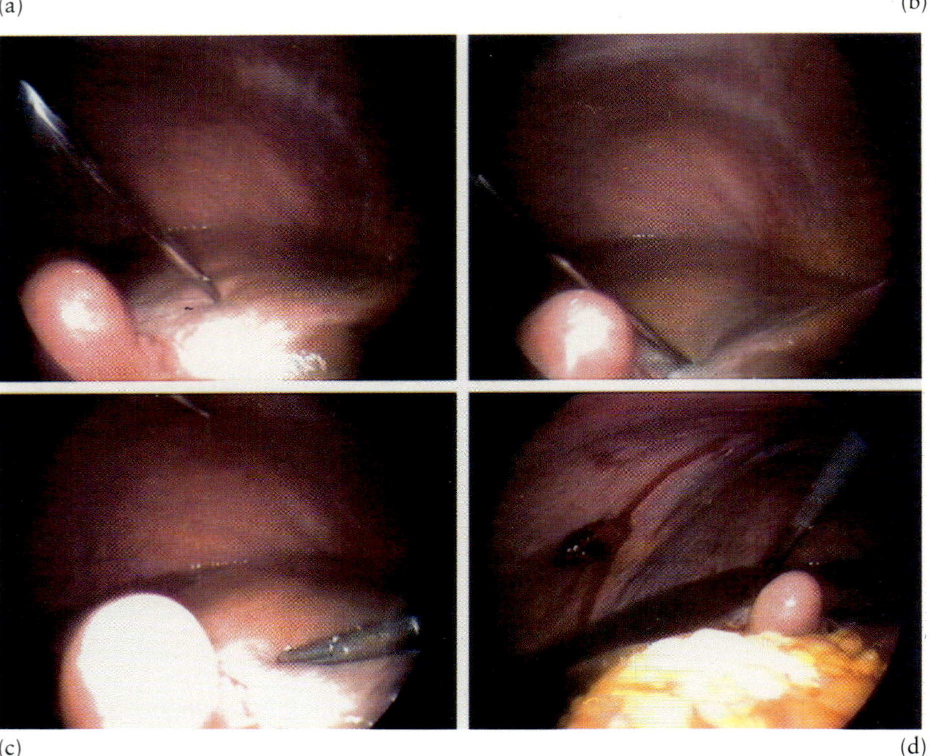

(c) (d)

Figure 2.5:   Core biopsy specimens can be taken with laparoscopic guidance, thereby assuring exact hemostasis. With either a spring-loaded or manual core needle: (**a**) the biopsy area is localized, (**b**) the core sample is taken, (**c**) pressure is applied with an instrument through an accessory cannula, (**d**) cautery is used as necessary to control biopsy site bleeding.

Special situations

Intractable ascites

It is not uncommon to find patients with tense ascites from either malignancy or hepatic cirrhosis. As with open surgery techniques, a major concern is the possibility of an ascitic leak in these patients. All medical attempts to control a patient's ascites should be thoroughly exhausted prior to operation. This includes vigorous fluid and salt restriction, diuretics and therapy specific to the disease process (eg chemotherapy).

To minimize the risk of an ascitic leak, to obtain a sample for cytology, and particularly to drain fluid to improve visual inspection, it is useful to use the shielded Verres needle for paracentesis prior to laparoscopy. This can be accomplished either at the time of operation or, depending upon the intent of the pathologist and anesthesiologist, at the bedside a day or two before the procedure. A minimum of 2 L of fluid removal is often required; therefore it is

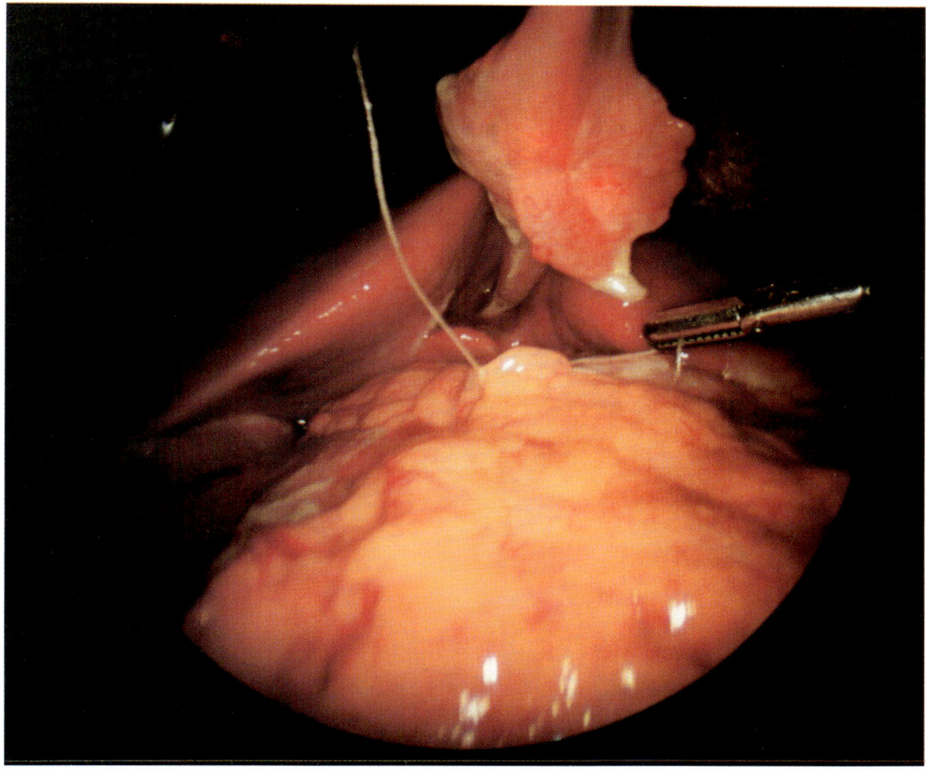

Figure 2.6:   Tissue biopsy specimens can be dissected with the aid of a suture placed adjacent to the mass.

Figure 2.7:   An inexpensive and ubiquitous specimen bag can be fashioned from any finger of a heavy-duty surgical glove. It is useful to cut the rim of this 'bag' so that a flanged opening exists with a longer tab on one side. This is used to facilitate grasping and positioning with laparoscopic instruments.

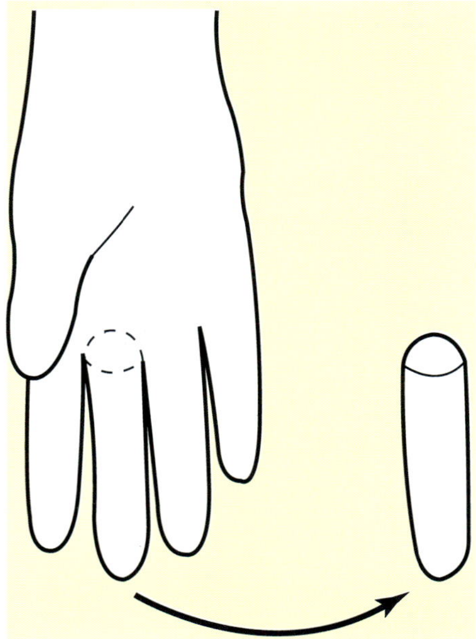

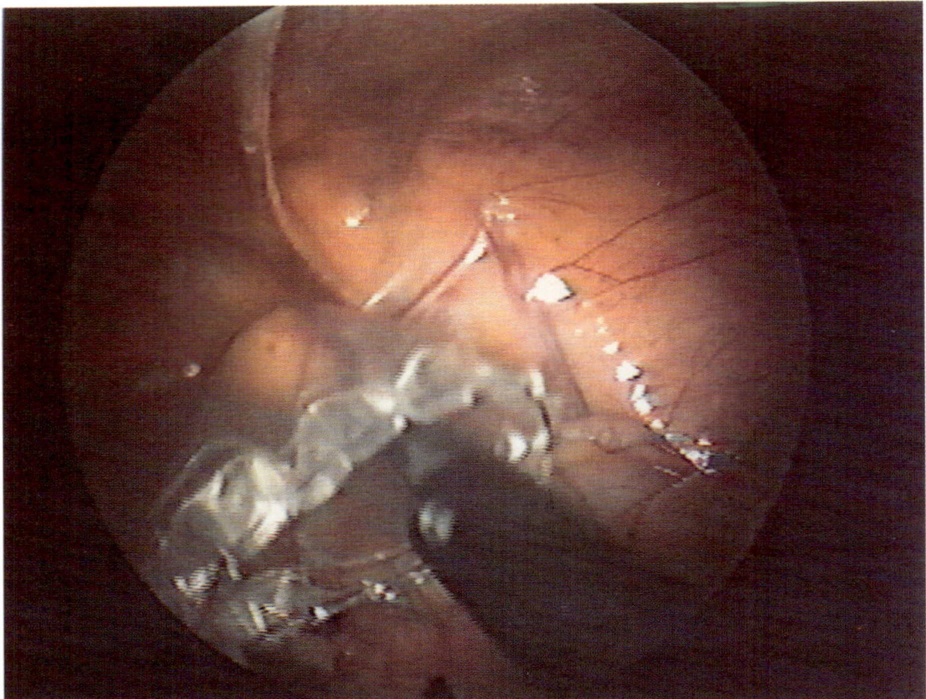

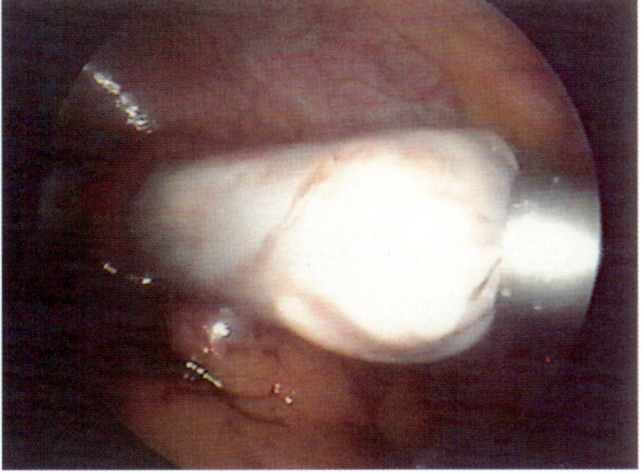

Figure 2.8: A specimen bag can be used not only for the temporary storage of multiple samples during dissection, but also to shield the abdominal organs from contamination by the specimen. Specimens are placed within the collection bag, and the neck of the sac is gathered and withdrawn either entirely or partially into the cannula. Withdrawing the bag/instrument/cannula assembly then leaves the neck of the sac outside the patient, and the specimen can be removed in pieces or the incision enlarged as desired.

crucial to pay close attention to the patient's postoperative fluid status and to measure urinary output.

The ascitic fluid that bathes the abdominal organs makes it imperative that exact hemostasis is achieved at operation. Not only is there no adjacent tissue to adhere to biopsy sites, but often it is just these patients that have significant coagulopathies. In addition, if there is portal hypertension, the risks of bleeding from biopsy sites increase substantially. However, it is precisely these patients who are at the greatest risk from other less invasive biopsy methods. These patients should specifically be considered for laparoscopic-directed biopsy.

To avoid a postoperative ascitic leak, it is critical to pay close attention to three methods of controlling ascites. The first is mechanical and meticulous closure of the abdominal wall in layers. The peritoneum is closed with a running suture, the fascial layers are tightly approximated with interrupted sutures and the skin is closed with monofilament subcuticular suture. The skin suture can usually be left in place for weeks with little concern of infection. Secondly, repeated paracentesis in the postoperative period may be necessary. This is easily accomplished at the bedside with a Verres needle under local anesthesia, and should be considered daily until the wound integrity is beyond question or the ascites is controlled. Thirdly, medical management of ascites with strict attention to fluid and electrolyte balance together with vigorous diuretic therapy. These measures will decease the pressure on the wound closure and thereby minimize the risk of an ascitic leak.

If these measures fail, one can attempt further bolstering of the wound closure at the bedside with wide mattress sutures, but one is well advised to return to the operating room for reclosure using all the equipment and facility of that environment.

Finally, if these conservative measures fail, a peritoneovenous shunt may be the only alternative to a prolonged ascitic leak, infection, further protein loss and other morbid complications. The possibility of needing a peritoneovenous shunt should be anticipated prior to the initial procedure and, if desired, directed placement with laparoscopic guidance is a simple adjunctive measure.

Coagulopathy

Uncorrectable coagulopathies represent one of the firm contraindications to laparoscopy. However, it is just this situation where, if laparotomy for biopsy or staging is required, laparoscopy may play a significant role. As with open surgery, electrocautery is liberally used when dissecting tissues. Complete hemostasis is assured with a rigorous inspection both during dissection and at the completion of the procedure.

Two situations unique to laparoscopy require special attention. First, most laparoscopic cases are performed with a positive-pressure pneumoperitoneum. This may limit the detection of venous bleeding from raw tissue surfaces, as venous pressure often approximates that of the pneumoperitoneum. Particular attention must be placed on all areas of tissue dissection, especially in patients with a coagulopathy. Secondly, the laparoscope cannula site is nearly impossible to assess for bleeding unless the laparoscope is placed through an accessory cannula. It is also useful to suture these sites under direct vision of the laparoscope (ie watching the passage of the needle with the laparoscope while the abdomen remains insufflated). When the laparoscope and instruments are then removed, there is no further trauma which can cause undetected bleeding.

Complications

Complications specific to laparoscopy can be divided into four main types:

- trocar and needle placement

- cautery or laser injury

- injury during dissection

- the effects of pneumoperitoneum.

The complication that is unique to diagnostic laparoscopy and laparoscopic-directed biopsy for malignant disease is tumor implantation at either the site of laparoscopic manipulation or at an accessory trocar site. This phenomenon has occurred following laparoscopy for gastric adenocarcinoma[21], after diagnostic laparoscopic biopsy of a serous ovarian tumor[22] and probably with many other types of malignancy that have not been reported. Every reasonable effort should be taken to avoid this morbid complication.

The future

Although diagnostic laparoscopy has been used in the diagnosis of malignant diseases for more than 80 years, it has found a welcome revival with improvements in optics and instrumentation over the past few years. The loss of tactile sense with laparoscopic surgery soon may be partially compensated for by the use of adjunctive modalities such as laparoscopic ultrasonography. Radioimmunologic-guided probes may also enhance detection of metastases and guide directed biopsy or staging. With rapid advances being made in areas such as gene therapy, laparoscopy may indeed play an expanding role in the diagnostic and therapeutic options for the victims of cancer.

Conclusions

Many patients with known or suspected abdominal malignancies will benefit from diagnostic laparoscopy with directed biopsy. This can either be done as the first step of a planned therapeutic procedure or staged separately days or weeks before resection. Minimal access techniques can also be used to perform a trial dissection to assess resectability or (in selected cases) to complete the therapeutic operation.

The current limits of these techniques are not due to the inability of laparoscopic tissue sampling or dissection, but result from the recognition by the clinician that this is a safe, accurate and particularly useful approach to patients with known or suspected malignancies.

References

1   Ott D (1901) Illumination of the abdomen (ventroscopy). *J Akush Zhenksk Bolez.* **15**: 1045.

2   Kelling G (1902) Ueber Oesophagoskopie, Gastroskopie und Kolioskopie. *Munch Med Wochenschr.* **49**: 21–4.

3   Jakobeus HC (1910) Ueber die Moglichkeit die Zystoskopie bei Untersuchung seroser Hohlungen anzuwenden. *Munch Med Wochenschr.* **57**: 2090–2.

4   Jakobeus HC (1911) Kurze Ubersicht uber meine Erfahrungen mit der Laparoskopie. *Munch Med Wochenschr.* **58**, 2017–19.

5   Bernheim B (1911) Organoscopy: cystoscopy of the abdominal cavity. *Ann Surg.* **53**: 764.

6   Kalk H (1929) Erfahrungen mit der Laparoskopie. *Z Klin Med.* **111**: 303–48.

7   Fervers C (1933) Die laparoskopie mit dem Zystoskope: ein beitrag zur vereinfachung der technik und zur endoskopischen Strangdurtrennung in der Bauchhohle. *Med Sche Klin.* **29**: 1042–5.

8   Ruddock JC (1937) Peritoneoscopy. *Surg Gynecol Obstet.* **65**: 623–39.

9   Benedict EB (1938) Peritoneoscopy. *N Eng J Med.* **218**: 713–14.

10 Verres J (1938) Neues Instrument zur Ausfuhrung von Brust oder Bauchpunktionen und Pneumothoraz Behandlung. *Dtsch Med Wochenschr.* **64**: 1480–1.

11 Hopkins HH (1953) On the diffraction theory of optical images. *Proc Soc Lond.* **A217**: 408.

12 Semm K (1978) Tissue puncher and loop ligation: new aids for surgical therapeutic pelviscopy (laparoscopy) and endoscopic intra-abdominal surgery. *Endoscopy.* **10**: 119–24.

13 Mackenzie DJ *et al.* (1992) Laparoscopic diagnosis of Ewing's sarcoma metastatic to the liver: case report and review of the literature. *J Ped Surg.* **27**: 93–5.

14 Easter DW *et al.* (1992) The utility of diagnostic laparoscopy for abdominal disorders. Audit of 120 patients. *Arch Surg.* **127**: 379–83.

15 Warshaw AL *et al.* (1990) Preoperative staging and assessment of resectability of pancreatic cancer. *Arch Surg.* **125**: 230–3.

16   Warshaw AL *et al.* (1986) Laparoscopy in the staging and planning of therapy for pancreatic cancer. *Am J Surg.* **151**: 76–80.

17   Hasan FA *et al.* (1989) Hepatic involvement as the primary manifestation of Kaposi's sarcoma in the acquired immune deficiency syndrome. *Am J Gastroenterol.* **84**: 1449–51.

18   Herrera JL *et al.* (1989) Diagnostic laparoscopy: A prospective review of 100 cases. *Am J Gastroenterol.* **84**: 1051–4.

19   Bhargava DK *et al.* (1992) Peritoneal tuberculosis: laparoscopic patterns and its diagnostic accuracy. *Am J Gastroenterol.* **87**: 109–112.

20   Warshaw AL (1991) Implications of peritoneal cytology for staging of early pancreatic cancer. *Am J Surg.* **161**: 26–30.

21   Cava A *et al.* (1990) Subcutaneous metastasis following laparoscopy in gastric adenocarcinoma. *Eur J Surg Oncol.* **16**: 63–7.

22   Hsiu JG *et al.* (1986) Tumor implantation after diagnostic laparoscopic biopsy of serous ovarian tumors of low malignant potential. *Obstet Gynecol.* **68**: 90–3s.

3

Laparoscopic staging of malignancy for the upper gastrointestinal tract and pancreas

FREDERICK L GREENE

Introduction

The role of the surgical oncologist in the management of upper gastrointestinal malignancy (including pancreatic cancer) involves surveillance, early diagnosis, surgical management and patient follow-up. Each of these phases depends not only on physical examination but also on new technology which allows enhanced radiographic and direct visualization of both the entire upper gastrointestinal tract and the abdominal cavity. As with the management of thoracic malignancy, the surgeon embarking on therapeutic intervention of cancer in the upper gastrointestinal tract, including the pancreas, must be familiar with endoscopic techniques. As thoracic surgeons have traditionally performed bronchoscopic examinations prior to definitive thoracotomy and lung resection, surgeons who manage gastrointestinal and abdominal malignancy should be responsible for endoscopic evaluation. The surgeon who manages malignancy of the esophagus, stomach and pancreato-biliary tract must appreciate the technical maneuvers necessary for laparoscopic visualization, as well as the interpretive skills that are necessary to make an early and effective diagnosis.

The American Cancer Society estimates that in 1994 there were at least 250 000 new cancer cases in the USA involving the digestive tract[1]. Of this number, there were 12 000 esophageal, 25 000 gastric, 16 000 hepato-biliary and 30 000 pancreatic carcinomas. In addition, deaths related to primary carcinomas of the gastrointestinal tract claimed 125 000 lives in the USA. 26 000 Americans died of pancreatic carcinoma while hepato-biliary, esophageal and gastric cancer claimed 13 000, 10 000, and 15 000 patients respectively. It is obvious that the incidence and death rates reported in the USA are lower than the total numbers of deaths expected in other areas of the world, including the UK and western Europe where incidence rates of pancreatic carcinoma are increasing. Similarly, there are areas of the world, including Asia and South America, where esophageal and gastric carcinoma continue to claim a majority of the population when gastrointestinal-related cancer deaths are recorded.

While laparoscopy has had a defined role in the diagnosis and staging of certain intra-abdominal malignancies such as pancreatic, gastric and hepato-biliary tumors, the excitement generated by therapeutic laparoscopic intervention has only recently been applied to the surgical therapy of gastrointestinal tract malignancy[2]. As technical innovation and physician expertise improve, diagnostic modalities of needle biopsy, lymph node biopsy, and direct visualization of metastases have given way to methods of extirpation of gastrointestinal tract malignancy, especially in the small and large bowel. Using diagnostic laparoscopy, a subset of patients may be identified who are more reasonable candidates for major extirpative surgery and who, in the long term, may not benefit from traditional open procedures. While the management of gastrointestinal tract cancer, such as carcinoma of the stomach and colon, continues to include attempts at palliative resection, future studies and trials will delineate the role of laparoscopy in defining groups of patients who may benefit from other multimodality therapies, thereby limiting the number of patients who must undergo extirpative procedures.

Evaluation and management of esophageal carcinoma

Throughout the world there is an increasing incidence of esophageal cancer. Despite new techniques for early detection through flexible endoscopy and the exciting prospects of chemotherapy in the management of patients with squamous cell carcinoma of the esophagus, the major deterrent to successful management of this tumor has resulted from late diagnosis and failure to biopsy small lesions because of the lack of appropriate awareness or suspicion by the examiner. Once the proper diagnosis is made, with endoscopic visualization and mapping of the mucosa both proximally and distally to the primary tumor, the usual evaluation for the assessment of regional metastatic disease must be undertaken using computerized tomography (CT), magnetic resonance imaging (MRI), abdominal ultrasound or nuclear medicine scanning. While these techniques are quite reliable, reports of their accuracy are based on indirect evidence and significant subjectivity by the interpreter of the imaging study. The advantages of laparoscopy in the management of patients with esophageal carcinoma are clear when direct evaluation can be made of the upper peritoneal cavity with the appropriate nodal dissection and biopsy as indicated. The following characteristics are associated with improved chances of survival: (1) tumors less than 5 cm in length, (2) no extent beyond the esophageal wall, and (3) the absence of lymph node metastases. In patients with one or more of the favorable predictors, only metastasis to lymph nodes and tumor penetration of the esophageal wall had a significant and independent influence on prognosis[3].

Although the best palliative treatment for esophageal cancer may be appropriate resection and reconstruction of continuity of the upper gastrointestinal tract, newer techniques involving non-extirpative methods obviate the need for major resection in patients who otherwise would not be candidates for extirpative therapy based on advanced local or regional disease. In a randomized study, Watt *et al.*[4] assessed patients with upper gastrointestinal tract tumors and showed that laparoscopy is more accurate than conventional CT and ultrasound for assessing the stage of patients with esophageal and gastric carcinoma. If alternative management involves laser ablation, endoscopic stenting and/or radiation therapy, along with newer chemotherapeutic techniques, it is then necessary to stage patients appropriately endoscopically because of the absence of tissue which may be available for pathologic staging using the TNM system[3].

The abdominal cavity is approached with patients under general anesthesia, preferably using a laparoscopic camera with both 0° and 30° capabilities. After the introduction of CO_2 to create a pneumoperitoneum, the laparoscope is introduced through the periumbilical region. Accessory trocars are positioned in the upper abdominal area which allow for appropriate mobilization of the lateral lobe of the liver as well as evaluation of the retrogastric and periesophageal regions (Figure 3.1). It is important to utilize existing imaging studies in order to make a decision as to the efficacy of laparoscopy in this setting. The definitive operative resection may be planned at the same time if laparoscopic evaluation reveals no obvious tumor in the upper abdomen. It must be remembered that upper esophageal, as well as middle-third, lesions may be associated with nodal metastases to the hilar area of the liver as well as perigastric and retroperitoneal areas. Although abdominal CT and ultrasound may miss these metastatic areas, subtle changes may direct the laparoscopist to search aggressively for positive areas of nodal metastases.

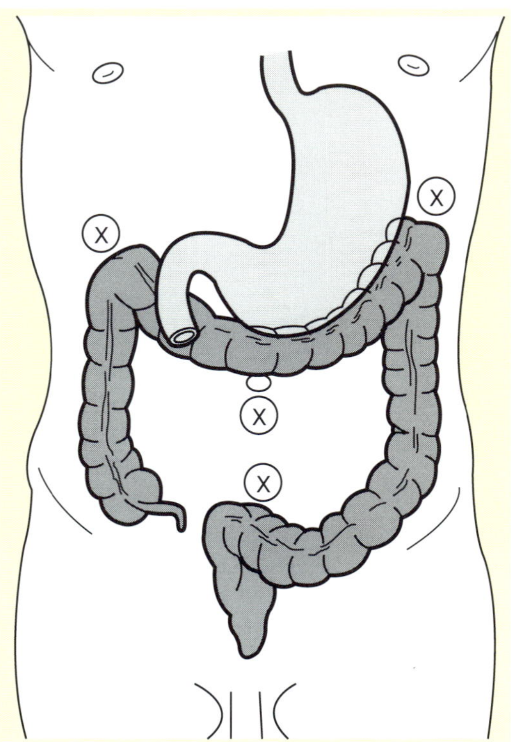

Figure 3.1:   Appropriate trocar placement for laparoscopic retroperitoneal inspection and nodal dissection.

Staging and management of gastric malignancy

Although the incidence of primary gastric carcinoma has fallen significantly during the last five or six decades in the USA, this tumor is especially significant in many areas of the world and continues to be a major risk in the Far East and Central and South America. The surgical approach to gastric malignancy has been similar to that utilized in the management of esophageal cancer, in that resection continues to be the primary modality even in cases of palliative management. Chemotherapy and radiation have failed to produce a reduction in the death rate from primary gastric tumor, and therefore surgical management continues to be recommended, especially when an advanced tumor is noted. Diagnostic laparoscopy just prior to abdominal exploration for gastric resection may be indicated in patients who have evidence on CT and abdominal ultrasound of advanced disease which may limit even palliative resection.

The approach to the abdominal cavity is similar to that used in diagnostic evaluation of esophageal carcinoma, but a heightened awareness of intra-abdominal metastases means that the surgeon-endoscopist must be careful in the initial introduction of pneumoperitoneum. An open technique, using the Hasson method[5], allows for the safe introduction of a blunt-tipped trocar and the eventual placement of both 0° and 30° laparoscopes and accessory trocars. Identification of perigastric nodes and exploration of the lesser omental bursa should be routinely accomplished in order to assess for fixation secondary to tumor or the finding of enlarged nodes which require biopsy (Figure 3.2). When

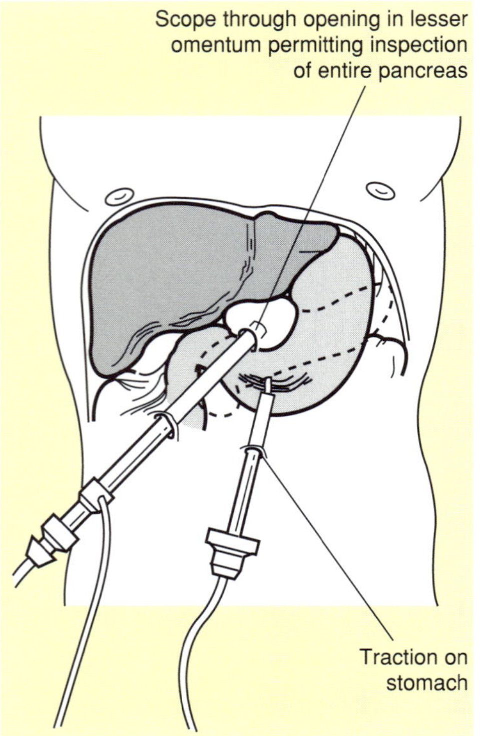

Figure 3.2: Laparoscopic approach to pancreas through lesser omentum or gastrocolic ligament showing alternative camera placement.

performing diagnostic laparoscopy, appropriate accessories must be available which include graspers, clip appliers, electrocautery probes and intra-abdominal retractors. It is especially important to be aggressive in the control of lymphatics and small bleeding vessels when nodal tissue is dissected. In addition, it is better to attempt resection of entire lymph nodes rather than to perform incisional or subtotal resection of node-bearing areas. This will provide the pathologist with adequate tissue for identification, especially if frozen section is being utilized before definitive exploration. The afferent and efferent lymphatics must be controlled to avoid the possibility of chylous ascites. Attention to detail is extremely important in order to reduce complications in patients who are not candidates for formal celiotomy. If intra-abdominal disease is noted, the placement of clips to outline the tumor may be indicated if adjunctive external radiation therapy is anticipated.

Laparoscopic staging in the management of pancreatic carcinoma

Adenocarcinoma of the pancreas continues to increase in both men and women. Unfortunately only a small percentage of patients are curable once the diagnosis has been made and appropriate plans have been developed for open surgical extirpation. While palliative resection for esophageal and gastric cancers may continue to have an important role, the routine use of pancreatectomy (whether subtotal or total) may not be appropriate if advanced local or regional disease is identified. The survival of these patients is limited to a few months once disease has been identified outside the pancreas, and therefore palliative measures such as biliary-enteric bypass of the obstructed common bile duct are indicated.

Studies have revealed that patients with pancreatic malignancy may in fact have early dissemination of tumor cells which can be discovered cytologically during laparoscopic evaluation[6]. The identification of occult pancreatic tumor cells provides the rationale for the poor outcome that may be noted after a potentially 'curable' pancreatic resection has been performed. Although visual inspection through the laparoscope is limited to the surface of organs, biopsy techniques with both needle and forceps can be used to assess tissue below the surface of the liver and within the retroperitoneum. Since pancreatic carcinoma frequently metastasizes to peripancreatic and perigastric nodes as well as the liver, biopsy techniques using both needle and forceps can assess tissue below the surface of the liver and within the retroperitoneum (Figure 3.3).

Although hepatic metastases are important sources of failure in pancreatic carcinoma, the real staging benefit for laparoscopy in this disease rests in the identification of surface implantation and the minimal ascites that may indicate a high likelihood of recurrence despite aggressive surgical treatment. Approximately 35–40% of patients with evidence of localized disease on conventional imaging studies may in fact have disseminated pancreatic carcinoma that will doom the patients to recurrence despite aggressive resection. Warshaw and coworkers[46] reported the evaluation of 88 patients deemed to be candidates

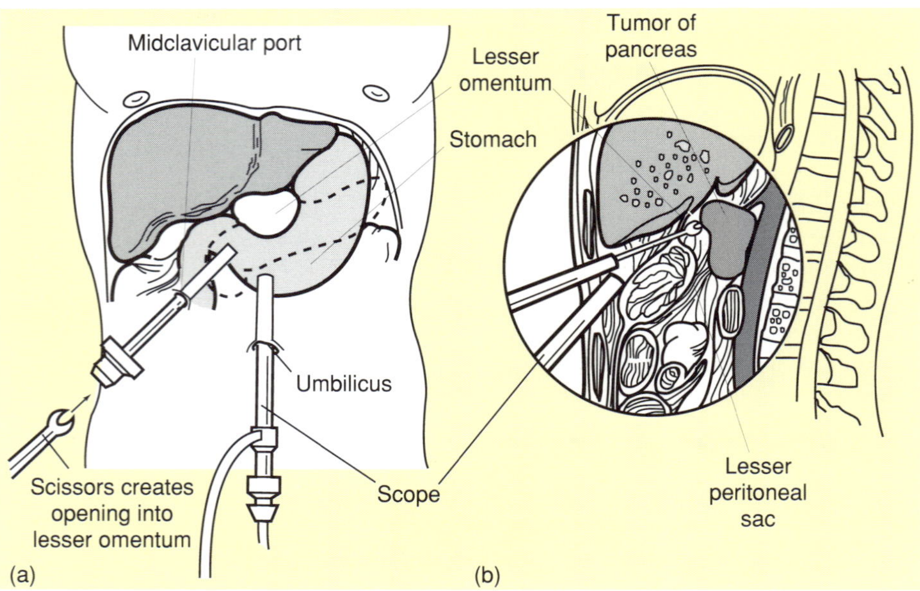

Figure 3.3: Laparoscopic approach to retroperitoneum through lesser omentum with approach to pancreatic tumor.

for surgery who had carcinomas of the pancreas or ampullary regions. Using CT, MRI, angiography and laparoscopy, 90% of the unresectable tumors were identified. Importantly, laparoscopy and biopsy enabled the identification of 96% of the patients who had small hepatic or peritoneal implants. These patients are much better served using palliative approaches to obstruction. Percutaneous or endoscopic stent placement may give the same long-term survival rate as traditional bypass procedures[7].

Techniques of percutaneous fine-needle aspiration and needle biopsy have been utilized to diagnose pancreatic malignancy. Laparoscopic examination and direct needle biopsy are safe and reproducible in the differentiation of masses in the pancreatic parenchyma. The surgical laparoscopist must be skilled in approaching the pancreatic body and tail through the division of the gastrocolic omentum or by entering the retrogastric space via the gastrohepatic ligament on the lesser curve of the stomach. Once these maneuvers have been learned it is possible to approach the node-bearing areas draining the stomach, pancreas and esophagus, and perform direct biopsy and partial resection of potentially involved nodes.

As a result of the advanced local and regional disease noted in patients with pancreatic carcinoma, the traditional role of the surgeon has also been to provide palliative bypass in patients with jaundice and pruritus secondary to hyperbilirubinemia caused by complete obstruction of the common bile duct. Laparoscopic maneuvers to achieve palliative bypass are now possible, and appropriate biliary-enteric anastomoses may be created without the morbidity created by large abdominal incisions[8]. In addition, gastrostomy or jejunostomy tubes may be placed to aid in the management of patients with extensive localized pancreatic carcinoma, thereby increasing the palliative role of laparoscopy as a therapeutic measure[9].

Contraindications and complications

The field of diagnostic laparoscopy should be subject to the same strict training, credentialing and privileging procedures as therapeutic endoscopic and laparoscopic techniques[10]. Improper selection of patients and poor technique may both cause problems. It has been shown that when proper teaching and adequate patient selection criteria are met, diagnostic accuracy is accordingly high, with sensitivity and specificity rates well above 90%[11]. The overall risk of mortality should be 0.1–0.2%, but this certainly depends on the patient's medical condition, which includes immune competence, nutritional parameters, evidence of sepsis and cardiopulmonary problems.

While some have advocated local anesthetic techniques for the management of these patients[12], we prefer general anesthesia because of the need for adequate pneumoperitoneum, and also the length of time that it may take to do an adequate staging procedure for upper gastrointestinal cancer or pancreatic neoplasia. Several studies have documented the cardiopulmonary consequences of the application of pneumoperitoneum, especially when patients are placed in the reversed Trendelenburg position for a long time[13]. It is important to monitor patients adequately and to assess the end tidal CO_2 levels closely throughout the diagnostic procedure. If patients are not suitable candidates for major abdominal exploration, they are unlikely to do well under general anesthesia for diagnostic laparoscopy. In addition to the assessment of cardiopulmonary function, careful assessment of coagulation parameters is important because of the need for concomitant liver biopsy, nodal dissection and biopsy of a tumor mass, which may be necessary during diagnostic laparoscopic procedures for malignancy. Although bleeding can easily be controlled with appropriate electrocautery and compression techniques, it is better to avoid biopsy initially in patients who have a prothrombin or partial thromboplastin time which in significantly altered.

Specific complications may occur from biopsy techniques of intraabdominal neoplasia. Abdominal wall implantation of tumor has been reported[14], and this may become more frequent as laparoscopic biopsy and therapeutic excision of abdominal tumors are performed. It is important to protect the abdominal wall as much as possible when performing either needle or forceps biopsy of tumors of the upper gastrointestinal tract and pancreas. This can only be accomplished by gentle dissection techniques and extraction of histologic specimens through appropriate trocar sites. By avoiding direct abdominal wall puncture and extraction of tumor through needle tracks, it is hoped that implantation of neoplastic cells can be avoided. Recently tumor implantation, even at the time of routine cholecystectomy, has become apparent because of the extraction of gallbladders that contain small cancers[15,16]. Since occult tumors will be identified in the biliary tree during otherwise routine cholecystectomy, it may be worthwhile to open the gallbladder at the time of removal to assure that carcinoma is not present. Although carcinoma of the gallbladder is not frequent, this neoplasm may in fact represent a significant percentage of carcinomas found in the upper gastrointestinal tract. Should incidental small cancers of the gallbladder be noted, excision of skin surrounding the port site may be helpful[17]. Exploration of the patient and excision of a portion of the gallbladder fossa may be indicated if a gallbladder carcinoma is identified[18]. More cases of tumor implantation will no doubt occur as more laparoscopic cholecystectomies are performed. It has been estimated that as many as one-third of gallbladders may have bile leak associated with extraction or dissection during laparoscopic cholecystectomy[19]. If so, it is obvious that small tumors of the gallbladder may result in peritoneal seeding or abdominal wall implantation; and as diagnostic laparoscopy is used more frequently for a variety of upper gastrointestinal tumors, there may be a concomitant increase in the number of later recurrences in the abdominal wall or peritoneum.

Future directions

Appropriate staging of gastrointestinal tumors depends upon providing adequate tissue to the pathologist at the time of surgical resection. In the future, with the growth of non-surgical modalities in the management of these patients, there will be less opportunity to stage patients pathologically, and therefore imaging techniques and laparoscopic nodal dissection will become more important as the primary tumor, nodal drainage areas and metastatic sites are assessed[20]. An even greater challenge to the surgeon is the use of the laparoscope as a means of applying radiation therapeutic and chemotherapeutic treatment to patients with these tumors. It is envisaged that radiation may be applied directly to the pancreas through the introduction of afterloading needles placed laparoscopically. In this manner, brachytherapy may be utilized to treat primary tumors as well as metastatic deposits in the liver. Similarly, if the current interest in cryotherapy for hepatic tumors continues[21] and is heightened by adequate outcomes, the probes may be placed directly, using the laparoscope to allow for freezing of tissue in a variety of intra-abdominal locations. Finally, the laparoscope may be a viable method for 'second-look' assessment of patients who are treated by non-operative means[22]. In order to reassess these patients, the surgeon-laparoscopist must become expert in the routine assessment of the intra-abdominal cavity and must be capable of assessing intra-abdominal tumor and retrieving tissue for full pathologic assessment. The applications of laparoscopy, both diagnostic and therapeutic, in the management of patients with abdominal malignancy of the upper gastrointestinal tract and pancreas will grow along with the growing creativity and expertise of physicians and instrument makers.

References

1   Boring CC *et al.* (1994) Cancer statistics, 1994. *CA Cancer J Clin.* **44**: 7–26

2   Greene FL (1993) Laparoscopic surgery in cancer treatment. In: Devita VT, Hellman S and Rosenberg SA. *Important Advances in Oncology—1993*. J.B. Lippincott, Philadelphia. pp. 157–66.

3   Demeester TR *et al.* (1988) Selective therapeutic approach to cancer of the lower oesophagus and gastric cardia: a prospective comparison for detecting intra-abdominal metastasis. *Br J Surg.* **76**: 1036–43.

4   Watt, I *et al.* (1989) Laparoscopy, ultrasound and computed tomography in cancer of the oesophagus and gastric cardia: a prospective comparison for detecting intra-abdominal metastasis. *Br J Surg.* **76**: 1036–43.

5   Hasson HM (1971) Modified instrument and method for laparoscopy. *Am J Obstet Gynecol.* **110**: 886–7.

6   Warshaw AL *et al.* (1990) Preoperative staging and assessment of resectability of pancreatic cancer. *Arch Surg.* **125**: 230–3.

7   Dowsett JF *et al.* (1990) Endoscopic endoprosthesis insertion following failure of cholecystojejunostomy in pancreatic carcinoma. *Br J Surg.* **76**: 454–6.

8   Shimi S *et al.* (1992) Laparoscopy in the management of pancreatic cancer: endoscopic cholecystojejunostomy for advanced disease. *Br J Surg.* **79**: 317–19.

9   Duh Q-Y and Way LW (1993) Laparoscopic gastrostomy using T-fasteners as retractors and anchors. *Surg Endosc.* **7**: 60–3.

10   Dent TL (1994) Credentialing and privileging for endoscopic and laparoscopic surgery. In: Greene FL and Ponsky J (eds) *Endoscopic Surgery.* W.B. Saunders, Philadelphia. pp. 499–507.

11   Spinelli P and Di Felice (1991) Laparoscopy in abdominal malignancy. *Prob Gen Surg.* **8**: 329–47.

12   Berci G and Cuschieri A (1986) Anesthesia. In: *Practical Laparoscopy.* Ballière Tindall, London. pp. 38–43.

13   Safran D *et al.* (1993) Laparoscopy in high-risk cardiac patients. *Surg Gynecol Obstet.* **176**: 548–54.

14   Cava A *et al.* (1990) Subcutaneous metastasis following laparoscopy in gastric adenocarcinoma. *Eur J Surg Oncol.* **16**: 63–7.

15   Pezet D *et al.* (1992) Partial seeding of carcinoma of the gallbladder after laparoscopic cholecystectomy. *Br J Surg.* **79**: 230.

16   Siriwardena A and Samarji S (1993) Cutaneous tumor seeding from a previously undiagnosed pancreatic carcinoma after laparoscopic cholecystectomy. *Ann R Coll Surg Engl.* **75**: 199–200.

17   Fligelstone LJ *et al.* (1993). Laparoscopy and gastrointestinal cancer. *Am J Surg.* **166**: 571.

18   Shiria Y *et al.* (1992) Inapparent carcinoma of the gallbladder: an appraisal of a
radical operation after simple cholecystectomy. *Ann Surg.* **215**: 326–31.

19   Fitzgibbons *et al.* (1993) Gallbladder and gallstone removal, open versus closed
laparoscopy and penumoperitoneum. *Am J Surg.* **165**: 497–504.

20   Greene FL (1993) Surgical endoscopy—a worldwide phenomenon. *Surg Endosc.*
7: 479–81.

21   Schneider PD and McGahan JP (1993) Percutaneous approaches to liver neoplasms. In: Hunter JG and Sackier JM (eds) *Minimally Invasive Surgery.* McGraw
Hill, New York. pp. 225–263.

22   Greene FL (1992) Laparoscopy in malignant disease. *Surg Clin NA.* **72**: 1125–37.

4

Laparoscopic staging of abdominal lymphomas

ALAN T LEFOR

Introduction

Lymphomas are a diverse group of malignant disorders of the lymphatic system that arise in nodal tissue and are categorized generally as Hodgkin's disease or non-Hodgkin's lymphoma. The treatment of lymphoma is dependent on the histologic type as well as the extent of disease. In most cases, treatment includes radiation therapy, chemotherapy or a combination of these. The role of surgery in the treatment of lymphomas is usually confined to obtaining tissue for diagnosis. In certain cases, usually involving lymphomas of the gastrointestinal tract, surgery is used as a therapeutic modality to resect the involved organ. This is often followed by chemotherapy and/or radiation therapy.

Invasive therapeutic and diagnostic maneuvers should be undertaken only when the results of such interventions will have a definable impact on the type of treatment given or on the course of the disease. Therefore the decision to undertake a surgical procedure for staging is made in consultation with the patient and the physician primarily responsible for therapy, usually a hematologist or medical oncologist. This is one of the few major abdominal surgical procedures undertaken strictly for diagnosis. It must be kept in mind that the use of laparoscopy to determine the stage of lymphoma does not influence the indications for the procedure or the components of the procedure, but only the specific technical conduct of the procedure. Furthermore, it is incumbent upon the laparoscopic surgeon to ensure that the procedure will yield the same pathologic material as if an open procedure had been performed; the diagnostic value of the procedure must not be compromised just so that laparoscopic surgery can be performed.

The surgical staging of lymphomas has undergone considerable evolution over the last 25 years. As recently as 1978, laparotomy was recommended for as many as 85% of patients with Hodgkin's disease[1]. With the refinement of noninvasive imaging techniques, as well as changes in the medical management of the disease, the subset of patients for whom surgical staging is necessary has become much smaller. This change in approach to the staging of lymphomas has significantly decreased the proportion of splenectomies performed for the staging of Hodgkin's disease. In a study from the University of Connecticut, 40% of splenectomies were performed for the staging of Hodgkin's disease between 1979 and 1985, while between 1985 and 1991, only 28% of all splenectomies were for the staging of Hodgkin's disease[2].

Laparoscopy has been used in the evaluation of lymphomas for many years. Laparoscopy was reported as early as 1973 in the evaluation of the liver in patients with Hodgkin's disease[3]. Bagley and coworkers reported in 1973 on 68 patients seen between 1969 and 1972 with untreated Hodgkin's disease[4]. Percutaneous liver biopsies to document subdiaphragmatic disease were performed first and, if negative, peritoneoscopy was performed. The presence of documented extraabdominal extranodal disease (eg bone marrow involvement) also eliminated the need for peritoneoscopy. Of the 68 patients evaluated, 12 has extranodal disease in other sites precluding the need for peritoneoscopy and nine were not further evaluated for other reasons. Of the 47 remaining patients, five had positive percutaneous liver biopsies and 42 underwent peritoneoscopy which revealed clinically undetected subdiaphragmatic disease in six patients. This early study at the USA's National Cancer Institute (NCI) concluded that laparoscopy could be an alternative to laparotomy in establishing the diagnosis of subdiaphragmatic disease necessitating treatment other than radiation therapy. Unfortunately the equipment available in the early 1970s was extremely basic compared with the advanced imaging equipment available today, and the role of laparoscopy was limited to establishing the diagnosis of advanced disease.

Non-Hodgkin's lymphomas

Non-Hodgkin's lymphomas represent a very diverse group of diseases with varied histologies and clinical courses. There have been a number of attempts to devise useful pathologic classification schemes and staging systems for non-Hodgkin's lymphomas. In general, it is not possible to use a single scheme for the staging of all patients with this very diverse group of diseases[5]. The most recent classification divides lymphomas into low-, intermediate- and high-grade pathologic groups according to the NCI Working Formulation[6], based on a comparison of six major classification schemes. Each of these groups is further subdivided according to cell type (eg small, large). The therapy for these patients is still in the process of evolution and surgical staging is reserved for a small minority at institutions where patients receive radiation therapy only for localized disease.

Staging evaluation of these patients is carried out in an orderly fashion once the diagnosis has been established by lymph node biopsy. A detailed history is obtained and a thorough physical examination performed evaluating lymph node-bearing areas. Laboratory studies including complete blood count (cbc), liver function tests, renal function tests, serum lactate dehydrogenase and alkaline phosphatase are obtained. Patients are then evaluated with imaging studies including abdominal computed tomography (CT) and Gallium-67 scanning in select cases. Bilateral iliac crest bone marrow biopsies are obtained as well. These will be positive in most patients with indolent low-grade lymphomas. Any patient with specific symptoms or signs of other organ system involvement are evaluated appropriately. Following this extensive evaluation, fewer than 20% of patients with indolent low-grade lymphoma of follicular center cell origin will require surgical staging of intra-abdominal disease[7].

The surgeon's role

The surgeon's role in the care of patients with non-Hodgkin's lymphoma is generally limited to biopsy of a single peripheral lymph node for diagnostic purposes. Abdominal surgery is rarely required. In patients with non-Hodgkin's lymphoma, laparotomy or laparoscopy may be necessary to obtain tissue for the diagnosis of intra-abdominal disease in the absence of peripheral lymphadenopathy. The limited use of operative staging of non-Hodgkin's lymphomas has resulted mostly from the improvement in imaging technology and other less invasive tests as well as the realization that precise definition of disease location, unlike that in Hodgkin's disease, has less impact on the therapeutic decisions to be made in these patients[5]. Laparoscopy may have a role in the evaluation of patients after treatment as routine imaging studies performed following treatment may overdiagnose persistent disease[5]. Staging laparotomy is restricted to those patients with clinically limited disease (stage I or II) who are to be treated using radiation therapy alone with curative intent[7]. In these cases, a staging procedure similar to that performed for patients with Hodgkin's disease (see below) may be undertaken laparoscopically. When surgical staging of abdominal non-Hodgkin's lymphoma is carried out, splenectomy may not be indicated since this will not often affect the therapy used[8].

Laparoscopy may have a role in the diagnosis of lymphomas which involve the gastrointestinal tract. Non-Hodgkin's lymphoma represents about 1–4% of all gastrointestinal malignancies, involving most commonly the stomach, but sometimes also the small bowel or colon. Patients with small bowel lymphoma typically present with a mass or obstruction. Complete, potentially curative resection is usually indicated, and if feasible, may be undertaken laparoscopically using laparoscopic tumor localization and bowel exteriorization with conventional bowel resection techniques. It is important to evaluate the entire small bowel since skip lesions may be present[8].

Colonic non-Hodgkin's lymphoma, when it occurs, often presents at the ileocecal valve. Intussusception is a common presentation, necessitating resection. Obstructive lesions of the distal colon also need to be resected. If the diagnosis can be made laparoscopically, treatment can also be performed laparoscopically. However, most patients who present with bowel obstruction are still explored with open laparotomy at our institution and the diagnosis of lymphoma is usually unknown prior to presentation. This may be a future role for laparoscopic techniques. Colonic non-Hodgkin's lymphoma presenting with diffuse submucosal disease is treated systemically and rarely requires resection.

The role of surgery in the treatment of gastric non-Hodgkin's lymphoma is still evolving. If resection is indicated and the surgeon is sufficiently experienced with laparoscopic techniques for gastric resection, then laparoscopy may have a role in the treatment of gastric lymphoma; at present this would be unusual.

Operative staging of most patients with non-Hodgkin's lymphomas results in upstaging a small number of patients usually from stage III to IV, due to occult liver involvement[5]. Since this does not change the need for chemotherapy, it is not usually warranted. If hepatic disease is suspected and its identification will impact therapy, then laparoscopy may be used to direct liver biopsy performed by percutaneous Tru-Cut needle (Baxter Healthcare Co., Valencia, California) or by wedge biopsy (see below).

In summary, the information gained from detailed surgical staging of patients with non-Hodgkin's lymphoma seldom has an impact on therapy and is therefore only very infrequently warranted. Laparoscopy may have a role in the diagnosis and treatment of some lymphomas of the gastrointestinal tract at this time.

Hodgkin's disease

Hodgkin's disease has been recognized as having a fairly orderly progression of disease since the description by Rosenberg and Kaplan[9]. In this landmark paper, they showed that Hodgkin's disease begins in a single nodal focus and then spreads in a predictable manner along adjacent lymphatic pathways. The Ann Arbor staging system has been used to describe the extent of disease in patients with Hodgkin's disease. In 1989 a new staging system called the Cotswolds Staging Classification (Table 4.1) was proposed, to reflect the widespread use of imaging techniques such as CT and magnetic resonance imaging.

A fairly standard evaluation is used for patients with Hodgkin's disease. The initial diagnosis can be made only by biopsy, usually of a lymph node since the disease most commonly arises in lymph nodes. After confirming the histologic diagnosis, a detailed history is taken, focusing especially on the presence of 'B' symptoms: night sweats, fevers and weight loss. A thorough physical examination is performed to evaluate node-bearing areas, together with laboratory studies (cbc, liver and renal function tests and serum alkaline phosphatase) and radiologic studies (chest X-ray, chest and abdominal CT scans, and bilateral lower-extremity lymphangiogram)[10]. While some claim that the usefulness of lymphangiography has been overshadowed by CT scanning, it does provide information complementary to that obtained from the CT scan, and both tests are usually obtained. Furthermore, lymph nodes which are abnormal on the lymphangiogram can be specifically identified in the operating room and biopsied at the time of surgery, unlike adenopathy seen on CT scan.

In patients with Hodgkin's disease, approximately 85% present with disease limited to lymph nodes, while only 15% present with extranodal disease as well[7]. In view of the orderly progression of disease along nodal groups, the need for surgical staging is more clearly defined in patients with Hodgkin's

Stage I:	Involvement of a single lymph node region or a lymphoid structure (eg spleen, thymus, Waldeyer's ring)
Stage II:	Involvement of two or more lymph node regions on the same side of the diaphragm (the mediastinum is a single site, hilar lymph nodes are lateralized). The number of anatomic sites is indicated by a subscript (eg II_2)
Stage III:	Involvement of lymph node regions or structures on both sides of the diaphragm: III_1: with or without splenic hilar, celiac or portal nodes III_2: with paraaortic, iliac, mesenteric nodes

Stage IV:	Involvement of extranodal site(s) beyond that designated 'E':
	
	A: no symptoms
	B: fever, drenching sweats, weight loss
	X: bulky disease:
	   > one-third the width of the mediastinum
	   > 10 cm maximal dimension of nodal mass
	E: involvement of a single extranodal site, contiguous or proximal to a known nodal site
	CS: clinical stage
	PS: pathologic stage

Table 4.1:   Cotswolds staging classification for Hodgkin's disease. (From Lister *et al.*[23], by permission.)

disease than in patients with Non-Hodgkin's lymphoma. The single determinant for the performance of a staging laparotomy is whether or not the information obtained will alter therapy. Those patients with pathologically documented disseminated nodal disease (stages III and IV) and those with pathologically documented extranodal involvement (eg bone marrow, liver) will require chemotherapy and thus need not undergo surgical staging[11]. Current treatment by stage can be summarized as follows.

Clinical stages I and IIA

Patients who present with a single site of disease high in the neck (ie peripheral IA) and have a negative imaging evaluation can be treated with radiation therapy alone, obviating the need for laparotomy. Those patients who relapse following treatment with radiation therapy alone are given chemotherapy without compromising the chances of long-term survival[11]. Patients who present with bulky mediastinal disease (greater than one-third of the greatest transverse diameter of the chest on posterior – anterior chest X-ray) are treated with combined modality therapy, making laparotomy unnecessary. Radiation therapy is not used on its own in patients with stage II massive mediastinal disease, since relapse rates of 50–74% have been reported[11]. The remainder of patients with clinical stage I/IIA disease require laparotomy if radiation therapy is contemplated as a single therapeutic modality, to ensure adequate pathologic staging of the disease.

Stage IIB

If patients undergo laparotomy and are pathologic stage IIB, subtotal nodal irradiation may be used. Clinical stage IIB patients who have not undergone laparotomy are treated with chemotherapy.

Stages III and IV

Patients almost always receive chemotherapy and laparotomy is not indicated.

Conclusions

A recent review of seven large series of routine staging laparotomy in the evaluation of newly diagnosed clinically staged Hodgkin's disease patients has documented upstaging in 25–35% of cases and downstaging in 5–15%[12]. Despite the accuracy of pathologic staging afforded by staging laparotomy, it is unclear whether staging laparotomy affords an overall survival benefit[13,14]. It is conceivable that most if not all patients who do not undergo surgical staging below the diaphragm could be 'salvaged' with chemotherapy if they relapse following mantle or extended mantle radiotherapy.

In summary, since a fair proportion of patients with Hodgkin's disease present with localized disease, and since Hodgkin's disease progresses in an orderly fashion, surgical staging to evaluate intra-abdominal disease is used much more frequently than in patients with non-Hodgkin's lymphoma. Prior to undertaking such a procedure, whether by conventional open surgical techniques or laparoscopically, it must be understood that the results of the procedure will impact on decisions regarding the therapy to be given. Patients who will receive chemotherapy, whether intra-abdominal disease is identified or not, are not candidates for surgical staging. Once it has been decided to stage the patient surgically, this can be successfully and thoroughly performed with laparoscopic techniques.

Surgical staging of lymphoma

The components of surgical staging for lymphomas have been fairly well defined[15,16], although there are some variations in the technique. Laparoscopic staging is best discussed in the context of the procedure as performed using conventional surgical techniques.

The procedure is usually performed through a long midline incision. Following thorough abdominal exploration, the liver is carefully palpated. Any abnormal areas are specifically biopsied. In the absence of specific lesions, a core biopsy of each lobe is obtained using a Tru-Cut needle; this is followed by a wedge biopsy of the free edge of the left lateral segment. The exact types and locations of biopsies are somewhat variable, with some authors preferring only wedge biopsies of the edge of each lobe without core biopsies. Since chemotherapy is indicated in patients with hepatic involvement, a frozen section diagnosis of Hodgkin's disease from an abnormal appearing area of the liver obviates the need for the remainder of the procedure.

The splenectomy should be performed next, especially in the absence of obvious hepatic lesions. The whole spleen must be removed and subjected to careful histologic examination as gross appearance is very unreliable. Preoperative administration of polyvalent pneumococcal vaccine is essential to lessen the risk of postoperative overwhelming postsplenectomy sepsis. Splenectomy is performed in the usual manner with careful attention to control of the hilar vessels and short gastric vessels.

The excision of representative lymph nodes is an essential component of the operation and must include a defined number of nodal areas. The random sampling of a few nodes is not adequate in the careful surgical staging of this disease. We routinely obtain a lymphangiogram preoperatively and are careful to biopsy any nodes felt to be 'suspicious' by their radiologic appearance. This is facilitated by the placement of clips at the site of resected nodes, after which intraoperative radiographs are checked to ensure that the resected node corresponds to the abnormal area seen on lymphangiogram. We routinely biopsy the following nodal areas: internal iliac (right and left), periaortic (right and left), portal, celiac, and mesenteric. Two things must be remembered when sending lymph nodes for histopathologic evaluation. First, the specimen should always contain an entire lymph node whenever possible. The structure of the node is important in establishing a diagnosis which is precluded by the examination of a nodal fragment. Secondly, lymph nodes should always be sent fresh in saline. The use of formalin prevents flow cytometric studies crucial to complete analysis of the lymphoma.

In young females who have not completed their families, oophoropexy is performed to help shield the ovaries from the radiation therapy which may be administered. While this does not guarantee maintenance of fertility, there is at least some hope for future childbearing. Shielding of the ovaries will help to maintain endocrine function of the ovarian tissue[8]. The ovaries should be marked with radio-opaque clips to help in planning the treatment fields. The procedure is completed by performing an iliac crest bone marrow biopsy which is draped into the operative field.

At the completion of the procedure, all operative sites are examined for adequacy of hemostasis and the packs are removed. The patient usually has a five- to seven-day hospitalization and is discharged with pain medications to be taken orally. Patients usually have four to six weeks of recuperation at home with limitations on physical activity, especially driving automobiles and lifting. They usually are able to return to work after this period. This recuperation time may also delay administration of definitive therapy.

Laparoscopic staging of abdominal lymphomas

The laparoscopic conduct of this procedure must not compromise the basic principles of this procedure described above. The indications for the operation and the components remain the same as though the procedure was performed using conventional open surgical methods. This procedure has been successfully performed laparoscopically by several groups[17,18], including our own[19]. This section describes a complete staging procedure such as that which would be used for Hodgkin's disease. Lesser or greater procedures may be indicated in the evaluation of abdominal lymphoma of the non-Hodgkin's type.

Our own experience with staging laparoscopy for Hodgkin's disease has resulted in the development of techniques to handle each of the component parts of the operation separately. We have developed extensive experience with laparoscopic explorations for a variety of malignancies with lymph node biopsies and specimen acquisition. We have also developed a technique for laparoscopic splenectomy which has become quite standardized[20] and can be generally carried out in less than three hours with little blood loss. In addition, we have developed a technique for the adequate laparoscopic wedge biopsy of the liver[21]. After extensive experience with port placement and operative techniques, we synthesized our knowledge into a single procedure which has allowed us to perform a complete staging operation.

The procedure is begun with the operating room set-up as shown in Figure 4.1. The operating surgeon stands on the patient's left side. Alternatively, the patient may be placed in modified lithotomy position with camera operator standing between the patient's legs. After insufflating the abdomen with CO_2, ports are placed as shown in Figure 4.2. We use 12 mm ports at all sites since the instruments often have to be moved from site to site depending on the anatomy encountered. The use of 5 mm ports would be unnecessarily limiting. An initial exploration is carried out looking for obvious lesions or areas of gross adenopathy.

The first procedure we perform is the liver biopsy. Any obviously suspicious areas are biopsied first (Figure 4.3), and frozen section analysis is performed since positive biopsies will eliminate the need for further intervention or biopsies. In the absence of any such areas, we obtain a Tru-Cut deep core biopsy

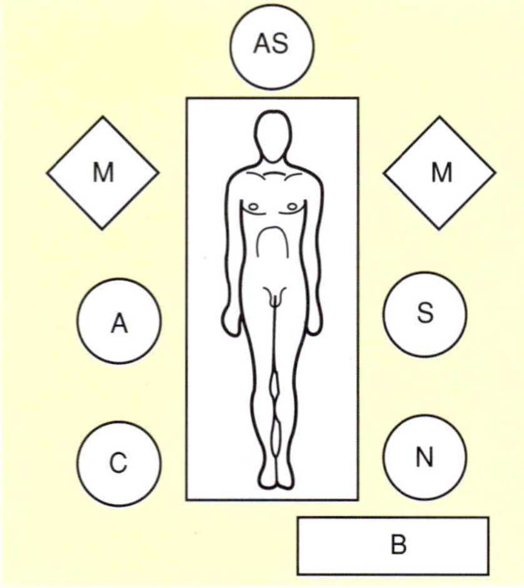

M: monitor/equipment cart
S: surgeon
A: first assistant
C: camera operator
N: scrub nurse
AS: anesthesiologist
B: back table

Figure 4.1:   Routine set-up of the operating room showing personnel position and monitor positioning for a laparoscopic staging procedure. The operating surgeon is on the patient's left side.

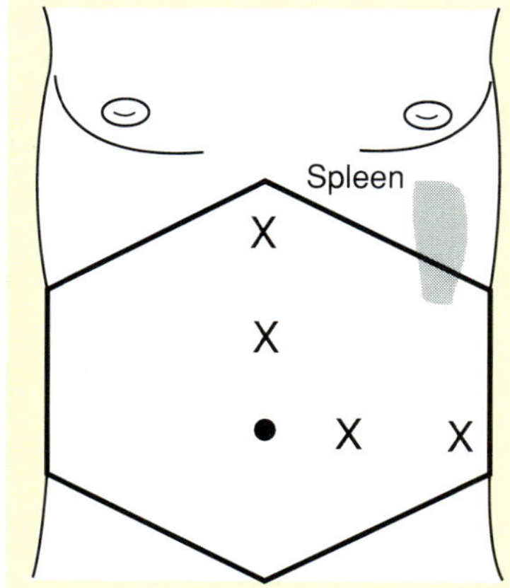

Figure 4.2: Port placement for laparoscopic staging of Hodgkin's disease. The midline ports are used for retraction and the left lateral ports are used for dissection and stapling. A sixth port may be necessary for dissection of the internal iliac nodes.

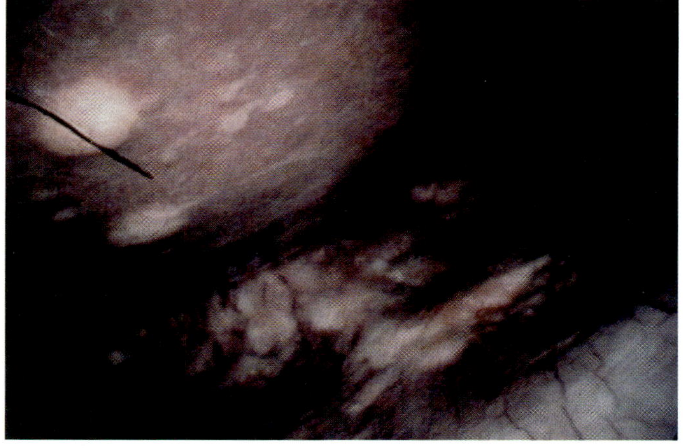

Figure 4.3: Directed biopsies are taken of any suspicious areas on the liver surface.

from each lobe using percutaneous introduction of the biopsy needle under laparoscopic guidance. We then obtain a wedge biopsy from the thin edge of the left lateral segment (Figure 4.4) using our previously described technique[21]. Briefly, the endoscopic linear stapler is fired twice at right angles to obtain a wedge of tissue and achieve hemostasis. While electrocautery could be used, it might destroy so much tissue that histopathologic evaluation would be adversely affected.

The splenectomy is performed next, and this is probably the most technically demanding portion of the operation. This procedure is described in Chapter 7, but a few details of the method developed at the University of Maryland deserve emphasis. We have not found preoperative splenic artery embolization—advocated by some[22]—to be necessary. The precise technique used to devascularize and dissect the spleen free from its peritoneal attachments is not important in the conduct of a staging procedure for Hodgkin's disease as long as it is hemostatic and safely executed. When performing a splenectomy for conditions such as immune-thrombocytopenic purpura one usually does not demand complete pathologic examination of the specimen; such is not the case, however, in Hodgkin's disease. Therefore morsellization of the specimen is unac-

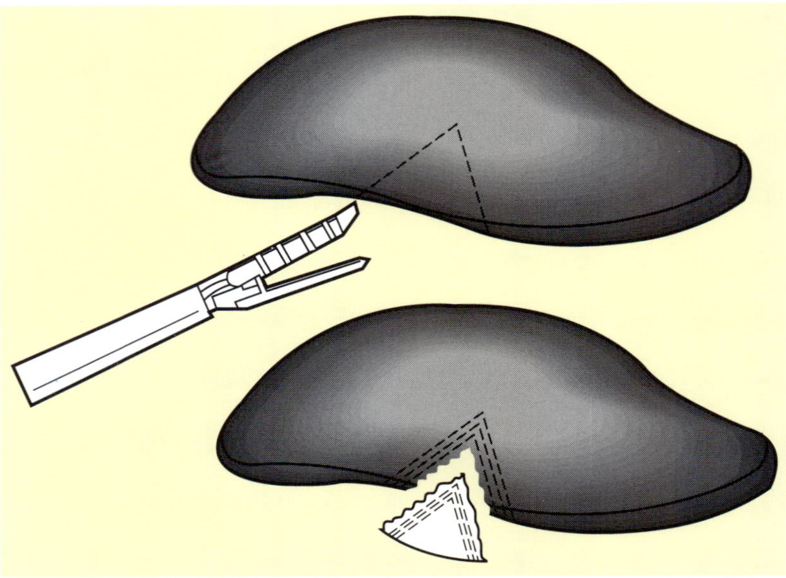

Figure 4.4:   The liver biopsy is performed first including needle biopsies of each lobe and a wedge biopsy of the left lateral segment with the linear stapler.

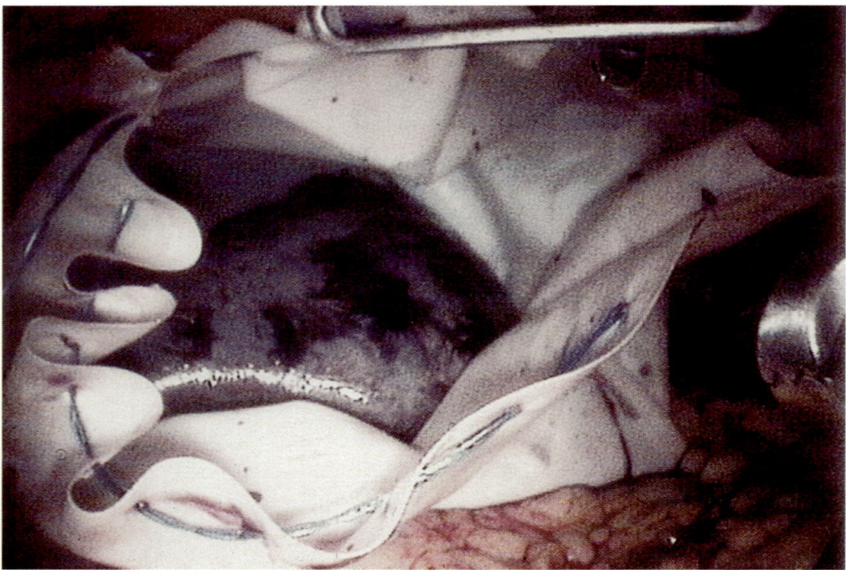

Figure 4.5:   After complete mobilization and division of the vascular attachments, the spleen is placed in a sturdy bag and left in the abdomen during completion of the remaining components of the staging procedure.

ceptable. We have chosen to use a stout plastic bag for removal of the spleen. The spleen is manipulated into the bag and left there for the remainder of the operation. The left upper quadrant is irrigated thoroughly with saline and the irrigant aspirated.

The lymph node biopsies are a challenging component of the operation when performed laparoscopically. As in open surgery, identification of nonpathologic lymph nodes can be difficult. This is made somewhat easier by the magnification afforded in laparoscopic surgery. The placement of an additional port in the lower abdomen may facilitate the dissection. One of the monitors should be placed at the foot of the operating table. The iliac nodes are approached first (Figure 4.6). The overlying peritoneum is sharply dissected away and lymphatic tissue can be identified adjacent to the vascular structures. Celiac nodes are approached after making a window in the lesser omentum superior to the lesser curvature of the stomach (Figure 4.7). A portal lymph node can also be sampled (Figure 4.8), and this remains perhaps the most difficult specimen to obtain. Identification and biopsy of mesenteric nodes is performed by sharply dissecting the peritoneum and careful dissecting in the mesentery. Periaortic nodes are also difficult to obtain and are approached in a manner similar to that used in open surgery. An alternative approach to mesenteric and periaortic nodes is to make a 6–10 cm midline incision at the end of the procedure through which the spleen can be extracted, and these nodal areas are directly biopsied. As with open node biopsies, any nodes that appear abnormal on the lymphangiogram should be specifically biopsied using intra-operative clips to mark the area, and using intraoperative X-rays to confirm that this is the abnormal node.

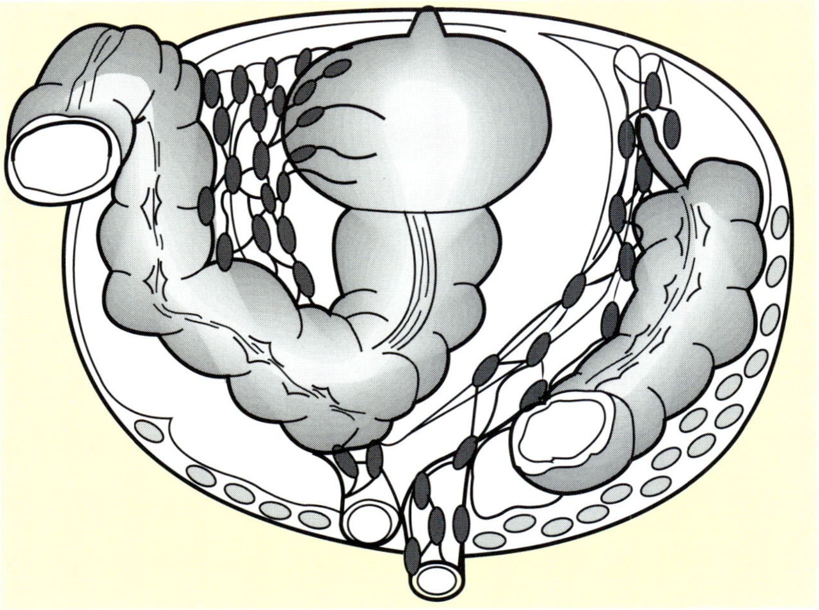

Figure 4.6:   The inguinal nodes are biopsied, obtaining a lymph node from each side. The nodes are located next to the iliac vessels and are dissected free from fibroadipose tissue after opening the overlying peritoneum.

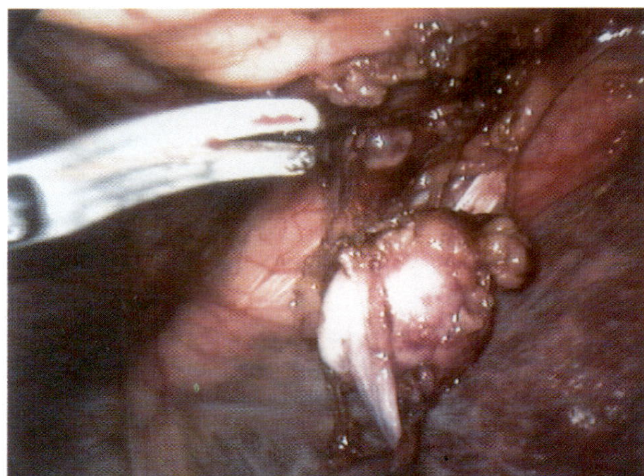

Figure 4.7: A celiac lymph node is biopsied after entering the gastrohepatic omentum revealing the celiac vessels with surrounding node-bearing tissue.

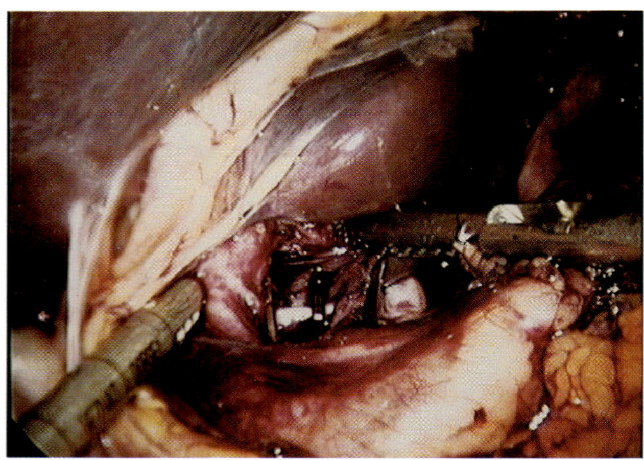

Figure 4.8: A portal lymph node is biopsied. The end of the suction tip (left) is on the hepatic artery while the grasper is in the lesser sac overlying the lesser curvature of the stomach. Nodal tissue is located next to the artery.

At the completion of all lymph node biopsies in young females, the ovaries can be sutured posterior to the uterus in an attempt to limit direct exposure to subsequent radiation therapy (oophoropexy). Clips are placed to help in planning radiation fields. Before ending the procedure, a bone marrow biopsy is obtained in the iliac crest using conventional techniques. The spleen should be removed intact through a small midline incision through which the open end of the bag is placed. An intact spleen is essential for adequate pathologic analysis of the specimen.

To date, there have been three cases reported in the literature of laparoscopic staging of Hodgkin's disease[17–19]. In one case, a 16-year-old underwent a staging procedure lasting 3.1 hours, including 28 lymph node specimens, multiple liver biopsies and splenectomy[17]. Estimated blood loss was 800 cc and the patients went home on postoperative day 5. Another 16-year-old underwent laparoscopic staging including lymph node biopsies and splenectomy[18]. This patient went home on postoperative day 3. A patient at our own institution underwent staging as described above[19]. The operation took four hours and the patient was discharged home five days later. He returned to work on postoperative day 11.

The laparoscopic conduct of this operation has several potential advantages to the patient including relatively rapid recovery time, decreased postoperative pain, and possibly earlier administration of definitive therapy. However, it remains a technically demanding procedure and one with which no single surgeon will probably gain vast experience. With advances in laparoscopic technology and refinements in techniques, the laparoscopic staging of Hodgkin's disease may become an important tool in the surgical armamentarium.

References

1   Bloomfield CD and DeCosse JJ (1978) Staging laparotomy. *Arch Surg.* **113**: 1135–42.

2   Marble KR *et al.* (1993) Changing role of splenectomy for hematologic disease. *J Surg Onc.* **52**: 169–71.

3   Casirola G *et al.* (1973) Laparoscopy in Hodgkin's disease. *Acta Hematol.* **49**: 1–5.

4   Bagely CM *et al.* (1973) Diagnosis of liver involvement by lymphoma: results in 96 consecutive peritoneoscopies. *Cancer.* **31**: 840–7.

5   Longo DL *et al.* (1993) Lymphocytic lymphomas. In: De Vita VT, Hellman S and Rosenberg SA. *Cancer: Principles and Practice of Oncology*, 4th edn. Lippincott, Philadelphia. pp. 1859–937.

6   National Cancer Institute (1982) National Cancer Institute sponsored study of classifications of non-Hodgkin's lymphomas. Summary and description of a working formulation for clinical usage. *Cancer.* **49**: 2112–35.

7   Williams SF and Golomb HM (1986) Perspective on staging approaches in the malignant lymphomas. *Surg Gyn Obst.* **163**: 193–201.

8   Palmer ML (1992) Surgical considerations in lymphoma. *Contemp Surg.* **41**: 13–18.

9   Rosenberg SA and Kaplan HS (1966) Evidence for an orderly progression in the spread of Hodgkin's disease. *Cancer Res.* **26**: 1225–31.

10 De Vita VT *et al.* (1993) Hodgkin's disease. In: De Vita VT, Hellman S and Rosenberg SA (eds) *Cancer: Principles and Practice of Oncology*, 4th edn. Lippincott, Philadelphia. pp. 1819–58.

11 Urba WJ and Longo DL (1992) Hodgkin's disease. *New Eng J Med.* **326**: 678–87.

12   Moormeier JA *et al.* (1989) The staging of Hodgkin's disease. *Hem Onc Clin NA.* **3**: 237–51.

13   Bergsagel DE *et al.* (1982) Results of treating Hodgkin's disease without a policy of laparotomy staging. *Cancer Treat Rep.* **66**: 717–31.

14   Taylor MA *et al.* (1985) Staging laparotomy with splenectomy for Hodgkin's disease: the Stanford experience. *World J Surg.* **9**: 449–60.

15   Grieco MB and Cady B (1980) Staging laparotomy in Hodgkin's disease. *Surg Clin NA.* **60**: 369–379.

16   Huang PP and Urist MM (1993) Evaluation of abdominal Hodgkin's disease. *Surg Onc Clin NA.* **2**: 207–11.

17   Carroll BJ *et al.* (1992) Laparoscopic splenectomy. *Surg Endosc.* **6**: 183–5.

18   Tulman S *et al.* (1993) Pediatric laparoscopic splenectomy. *J Ped Surg.* **28**: 689–92.

19   Lefor AT *et al.* (1993) Laparoscopic staging of Hodgkin's disease. *Surg Onc.* **2**: 217–20.

20   Lefor AT *et al.* (1993) Laparoscopic splenectomy in the management of immune thrombocytopenic purpura. *Surgery.* **114**: 613–18.

21   Lefor AT and Flowers JL. (1994) Laparoscopic wedge biopsy of the liver. *J Am Coll Surg.* **178**: 307–8.

22   Poulin E *et al.* (1993) Laparoscopic splenectomy: clinical experience and the role of preoperative splenic artery embolization. *Surg. Lap Endosc.* **3**: 445–50.

23   Lister TA *et al.* (1989) Report of a committee convened to discuss the evaluation and staging of patients with Hodgkin's disease: Cotswald meeting. *J Clin Onc.* **7**: 1630–6.

5

Techniques of abdominal lymph node evaluation, biopsy and dissection

THOMAS A STELLATO

Historical introduction

In the preface of his masterful treatise on *The Lymphatics in Cancer*, CD Haagensen quoted Lord Moynihan who in 1908 stated that 'the surgery of malignant disease is not the surgery of organs, it is the anatomy of the lymphatic system'[1]. Although currently the utility of therapeutic lymphatic dissection for some cancers is being questioned, the importance of evaluating lymph node involvement for staging (diagnosis) remains unchallenged. Prior to the development of sophisticated imaging techniques such as ultrasound and computerized tomography (CT), evaluation of the lymphatic system relied upon the injection of vital dyes into subcutaneous tissues. The technique of lymphangiography was devised by Kinmouth in 1952[2,3]. By injecting patent blue violet into the subcutaneous tissues and muscles of the hand or foot, lymphatic trunks could be visualized. An individual trunk would then be dissected, cannulated and injected with a water-soluble radiopaque contrast medium to produce a radiograph of the lymphatic vessels.

The technique described by Kinmouth formed the basis for lymphangiography; however, the transition in the 1960s from water-soluble contrast media to oily contrast media which do not mix with lymph expanded the diagnostic potential of lymphangiography[4]. The latter enabled visualization of lymph nodes and lymphatics of the thorax, abdomen and pelvis (Figure 5.1). Although spectacular radiographic images of the lymphatic system can be obtained with lymphangiography, the demands of the technique, the difficulty of interpretation and the development of other noninvasive imaging modalities diminished the importance of the lymphangiogram.

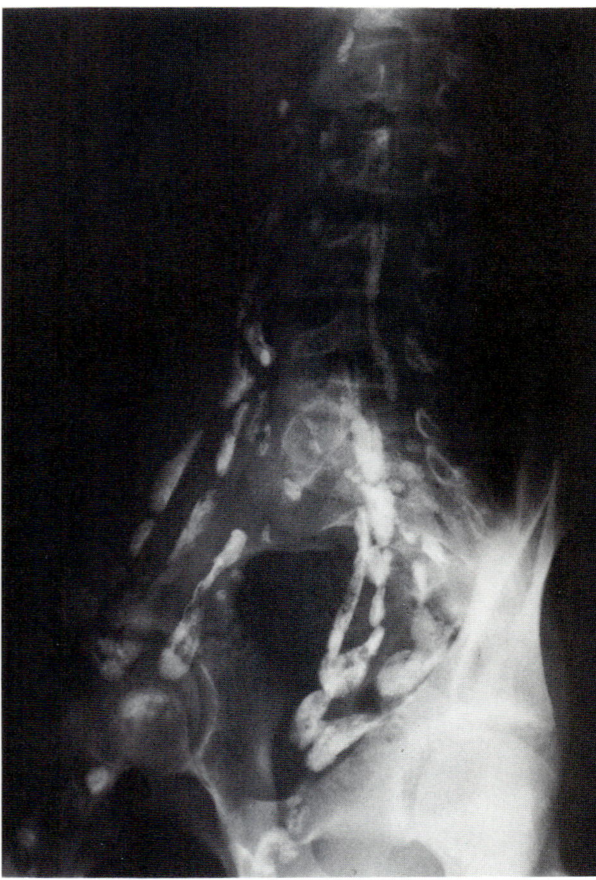

Figure 5.1: Normal lymph-angiogram. (Courtesy of John Haaga MD, Chairman of Radiology, University Hospitals of Cleveland.)

Lymph node evaluation

Noninvasive techniques like abdominal and pelvic ultrasound and CT, and more recently endoscopic ultrasound (EUS), can be used to identify lymph node abnormalities, and may possibly also provide the means for directed biopsy. Evaluation of lymph nodes by CT relies mainly on enlargement of individual nodes or groups of nodes (Figure 5.2). Although this imaging modality is relatively sensitive for identifying lymph node enlargement (lymph-adenopathy), its specificity in correctly differentiating malignant nodal involvement from non-pathology is relatively low. Lymph nodes involved in metastasis may be normal in size, enlarged or totally replaced by tumor. Although CT-guided needle aspiration cytology or needle biopsy may be extremely valuable in non-lymphomatous malignancies metastatic to lymph nodes, this technique is usually inadequate to confirm the diagnosis of lymphoma (Figure 5.3).

Ultrasound is less expensive than CT for lymph node evaluation, but both the attainment and interpretation of ultrasound images is much more technically demanding than CT scanning. EUS combines the technology of ultrasound with the ability of flexible endoscopy to truncate distances between the

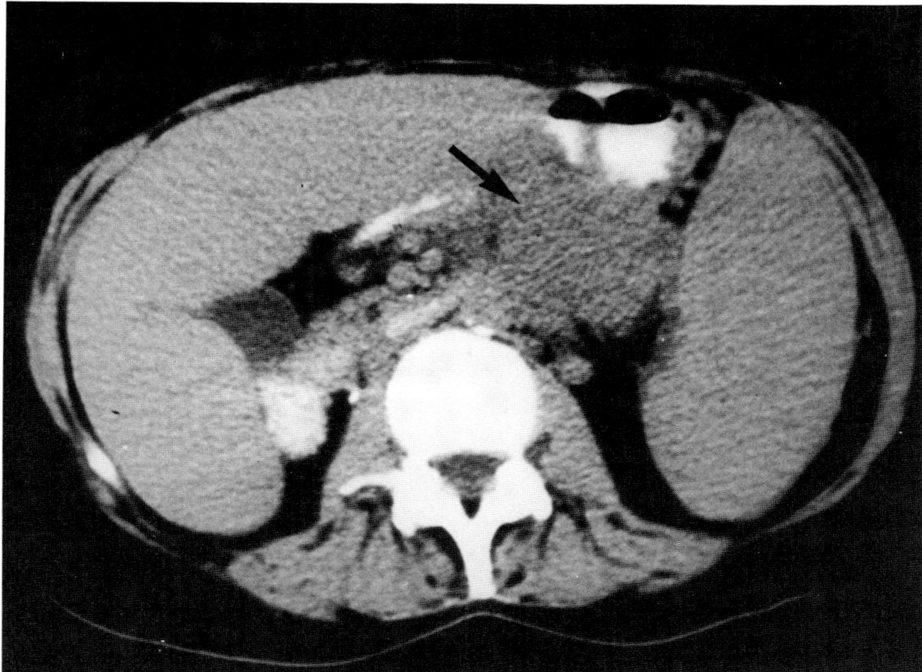

Figure 5.2:   CT scan of 54-year-old female with large retrogastric mass (*arrow*) consistent with adenopathy.

ultrasound transducer and the tissue under investigation. Theoretically this improves resolution and accuracy of the ultrasound examination. EUS has provided information regarding rectal cancer and upper gastrointestinal malignancies including those of the esophagus, stomach, duodenum and pancreas. Lymph node involvement by cancer is identified as a hypoechoic echopattern. Lymph node size has been directly correlated with tumor involvement in patients with rectal cancer examined by ultrasound (53.8% when nodes had a diameter greater than 5 mm vs 15.2% when nodes were not demonstrated by ultrasound or were less than 4 mm). Additionally, when nodes had an ill defined boundary but an even hyperechoic intranodal pattern, metastases were identified in 18.4%, while in nodes with a well defined boundary but an uneven and markedly hypoechoic intranodal pattern the incidence of nodal metastasis was 72.3%[5].

One of the newest technologies for identifying malignancy and nodal metastasis is positron emission tomography (PET) scanning. PET scanning measures the metabolic activity of malignant tissue by the incorporation of a radiolabeled metabolite. Since neoplastic tissue has an increased metabolic rate with increased glycolysis and lactate production, fluorine 18-labeled deoxyglucose (FDG) injected intravenously can differentiate malignant from nonmalignant tissue by PET evaluation[6] (Figure 5.4).

All of the above, lymphangiography, CT, transcutaneous ultrasound, EUS and PET, provide indirect information regarding lymph node involvement by malignancy with varying accuracy. Other modalities such as magnetic resonance imaging (MRI) and radiolabeled antibody scanning may also

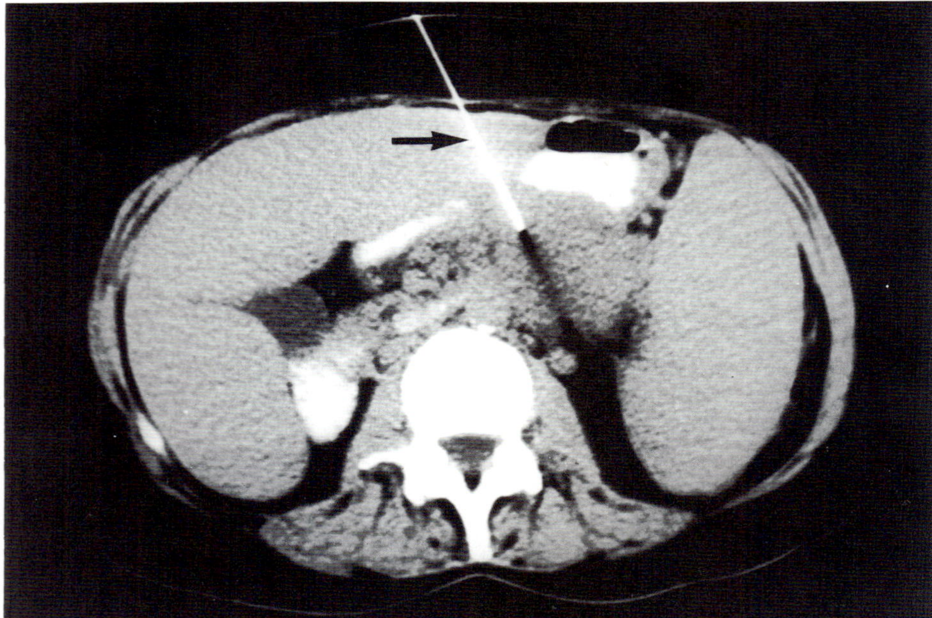

Figure 5.3:   Same patient as in Figure 5.2. CT-directed biopsy of retroperitoneal mass. Despite excellent positioning of the needle (*arrow*), biopsy was nondiagnostic. Patient underwent laparoscopic evaluation and biopsy. Results indicated that the mass represented large cell lymphoma.

provide similar information. However, most therapeutic decisions are based not on indirect information but on histopathologic information which requires direct access to lymph nodes. The above modalities may eventually be refined to the degree that they obviate histopathologic correlation, but at present they more often provide us with a 'road-map' to guide us in our biopsy or lymph-adenectomy.

Laparoscopic evaluation

In 1978, Meyer-Burg and Ziegler published the first report specifically address-ing the laparoscopic inspection and biopsy of abdominal lymph nodes[7]. They noted that there were only two earlier mentions of lymph node evaluation during laparoscopy. An atlas of laparoscopy authored by Kalk and Wildhirt in 1962 concluded that normal lymph nodes were rarely visible but lymph-adenopathy secondary to tuberculosis or malignancy could sometimes be identified in the region of the greater curvature of the stomach[8]; and Beck's atlas of laparoscopy from 1968 reported that enlarged lymph nodes from Crohn's disease might be visualized laparoscopically[9].

Meyer-Burg and Ziegler reported that normal gastric lymph nodes can be identified especially if patients are not obese[7]. These nodes range in size from 0.2 to 1 cm and appear as brown and red flat discs. The color is important, since both lymph nodes and the pancreas have a glandular structure but the pancreas is usually white or yellow in color. They also stated that nodes up to

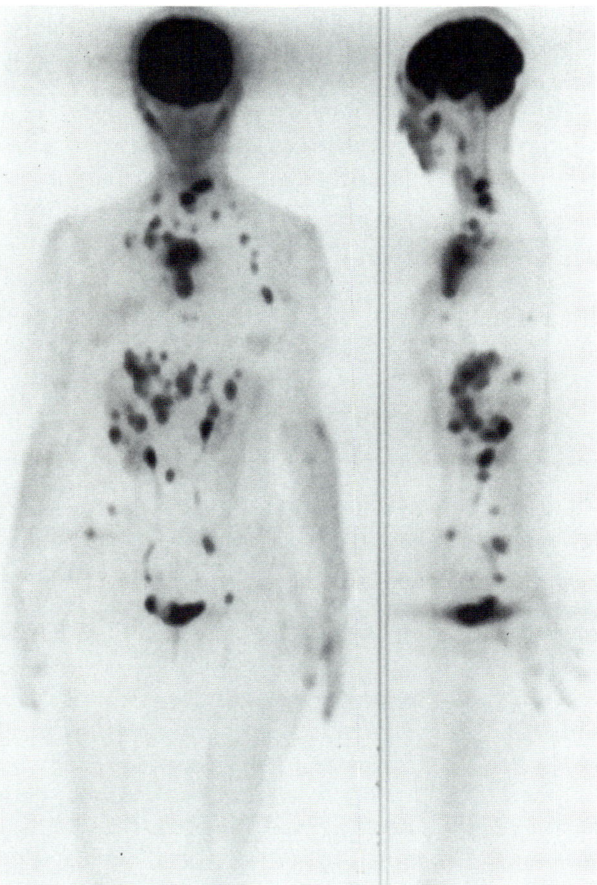

Figure 5.4: Positron emission tomography scan (mobile PET, Siemmens ECAT/EXACT 47-slice whole-body PET scanner) using FDG. This patient with known breast cancer shows multiple nodes and strong uptake in the manubrium. Bone scan did not become positive until five months after the PET scan. (Courtesy of Floro Miraldi MD, Chief of Nuclear Medicine, University Hospitals of Cleveland.)

5 cm and greater were usually associated with pathologic conditions. The technique necessary to visualize these nodes requires that the patient be placed on his right side with the head of the table raised and the left lobe of the liver elevated. The authors also reported the ability to 'biopsy' these nodes; their description is that of needle aspiration cytology and represents one of the earliest publications of laparoscopic cytologic lymph node evaluation.

Retroperitoneal evaluation

Retroperitoneal evaluation by laparoscopy is a relatively recent development. In 1988, Salky and colleagues from Mount Sinai Hospital in New York reported their experience with 19 patients over a five-year period in whom the primary indication for laparoscopy was retroperitoneal disease[10]. In each patient the retroperitoneal process had been identified by CT scanning. Laparoscopic biopsies were taken using a Tru-Cut needle or a lancet-shaped biopsy forceps. A positive biopsy and diagnosis were obtained in 17 of the 19 patients; 10 patients had lymphoma identified and 16 of the 19 patients were spared a laparotomy. Success in performing the retroperitoneal biopsy was related to two factors: (1) patients who had palpable retroperitoneal processes, and (2) noninvasive studies such as CT or barium contrast indicating the displacement of some viscus by the retroperitoneal process. Therefore the authors made a conclusion which is no longer valid: that patients with minimal retroperitoneal adenopathy seen by CT were not candidates for laparoscopic evaluation. They emphasized the importance of laparoscopic core needle or forceps biopsy when the diagnosis of lymphoma was entertained in order to maintain lymphatic architecture, as well as to provide adequate tissue for tumor markers.

Lymph node biopsy and dissection

As noted above, the sampling by core needle or biopsy forceps of both intra-abdominal and retroperitoneal lymph nodes, while far from routine, had proved feasible by the late 1980s. These techniques can provide large samples of lymph node tissue for histopathology as well as immunochemistry. As with open lymph node biopsy, the disruption of the lymph node in performing an 'incisional' biopsy, especially with biopsy forceps, almost always produces bleeding and requires some mechanism of hemostasis. While forceps are available which can allow coagulation while the biopsied tissue is still present in the forceps, coagulation in this manner can produce artifact as well decreasing the amount of tissue available for pathologic inspection. When using core needle or cup biopsy forceps, my preferred technique is to obtain the tissue and then apply coagulation with a specifically designed coagulation instrument such as the laparoscopic spatula (Figure 5.5). This instrument also allows irrigation. The technique for obtaining hemostasis should not be haphazard. Once the biopsy is taken, the spatula is applied to the biopsied surface. If the position of the spatula is correct, pressure from the spatula will arrest any

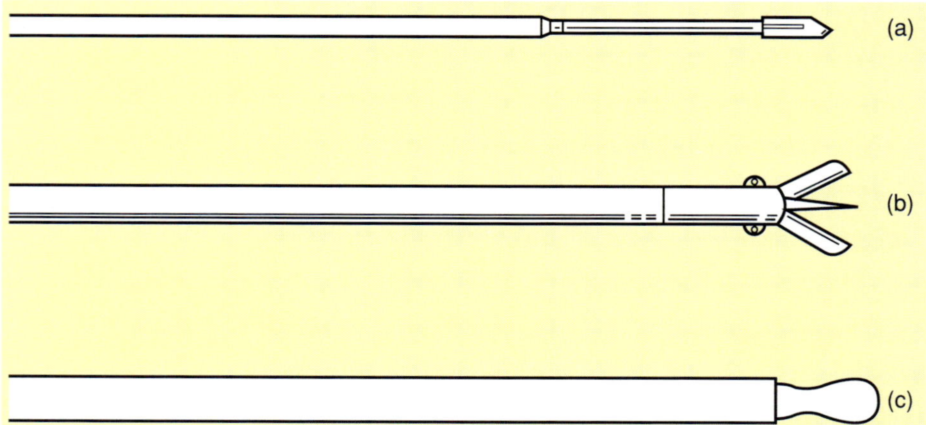

Figure 5.5:   Instruments for lymph node biopsy and hemostasis. (a) core needle biopsy, (b) spike-cup biopsy forceps, (c) laparoscopic spatula with irrigation channel.

bleeding. If bleeding continues, the spatula should be repositioned until optimal placement is found, so that the pressure from the spatula tamponades the bleeding. Irrigation can then be performed to clear the field of residual blood. Only then should coagulation by applied. This technique avoids unnecessary coagulation and necrosis to tissue which is not contributing to the bleeding.

The progression from laparoscopic lymph node biopsy to lymph node excision and dissection occurred concurrently with the development of other aspects of operative laparoscopy. A variety of factors contributed to this evolution, including the greater application of laparoscopy, improvements in instrumentation, growing operative expertise, and the development of video-laparoscopy. The time from the inception of laparoscopy in 1902 to the arrival of videolaparoscopy in the 1980s was characterized by slow and steady growth, unlike the dramatic advances which videolaparoscopy has brought about[11]. There is little doubt that the use of microchip cameras with laparoscopy facilitated the advances from simple to more complex operative laparoscopic procedures.

Lymph node biopsy by core needle or forceps provides a portion of the lymph node and requires hemostasis of the cut or torn surface. This is in distinction to lymph node excision. Laparoscopic lymph node excision is performed using atraumatic grasping forceps to elevate the node and identify its lymphovascular connections which are clipped, tied or coagulated, thus providing an intact lymph node in a more controlled fashion. We have used this technique laparoscopically to sample portahepatis lymph nodes in patients with hepatoma prior to chemotherapy treatment and subsequent hepatic transplantation.

Lymphadenectomy

The advancement from laparoscopic lymph node excision to lymph node dissection (lymphadenectomy) focused on pelvic malignancies. Dargent and Salvat from France introduced a retroperitoneal endoscopic approach to lymphadenectomy in 1988[12]. 'Pelviscopie retroperitoneale panoramique' (PRPP) entailed inserting the laparoscope beneath the deep fascia through a midline incision at the pubis. Although most subsequent interest was directed towards the transperitoneal (rather than retro- or extraperitoneal) approach to the retroperitoneal lymph nodes, there has also been continued interest in extraperitoneal endoscopic dissection. Pelvic lymphadenoscopy has been de-scribed by the extraperitoneal approach through a small oblique iliac incision without carbon dioxide insufflation. Taillandier and associates[13] reported 78 such lymphadenoscopies in 48 patients (40 with prostate cancer and eight with bladder cancer). Twenty three patients had unexpected lymph node metastasis (CT was considered normal). Extraperitoneal laparoscopic pelvic lymph-adenectomy utilizing low-pressure carbon dioxide insufflation has been com-pared with laparoscopic transperitoneal lymph node dissection in the staging of prostate and bladder cancer[14]. Morbidity was decreased with the extraperi-toneal approach, which subjectively seemed to be better tolerated.

Familiarity with intra-abdominal and retroperitoneal anatomy from experience during celiotomy and laparoscopy is probably the most significant explanation for the predominant focus on the transperitoneal approach to laparoscopic lymph node dissection. In 1988, Reich and colleagues reported one of the first transperitoneal laparoscopic pelvic lymphadenectomies for the staging of ovarian cancer[15]. This case report was quickly followed by reports of laparoscopic pelvic lymph node dissection in staging cancer of the cervix[16,17]. The laparoscopic approach means that a radical hysterectomy does not have to be performed when metastatic nodes are identified.

The potential advantage of avoiding radical prostate extirpation when positive lymph nodes are present provided a similar incentive for the development of laparoscopic pelvic lymph node dissection for prostate cancer[18,19] (Figures 5.6–5.8). A comparison between open pelvic lymphadenectomy and laparoscopic technique in patients with prostate cancer identified no significant difference in the number of lymph nodes removed (11 ± 5.7 vs 10.7 ± 5.7)[20]. Metastasis to lymph nodes occurs more commonly on the side of the pelvis which is ipsilateral to the side of the prostate where the lesion resides[21]. This information should direct the surgeon to approach the initial pelvic lymph node dissection ipsilateral to the side of the palpable prostate tumor. The accumulated experience of eight medical centers performing laparoscopic pelvic lymph node dissection reported a complication rate of 15% (55 complications in 372 patients)[22]. Complications included 11 vascular injuries, eight viscus injuries, 10 genitourinary problems, seven functional or mechanical bowel obstructions, five cases of deep vein thrombosis, five infections, five cases of lymphedema and two obturator nerve palsies. The authors concluded that there is a significant learning curve with this procedure.

Laparoscopic retroperitoneal lymphadenectomy beyond the pelvis to the para-aortic nodes has been performed in one patient with testicular cancer and another with carcinoma of the cervix[23,24]. In the latter case, this was performed concomitantly with a laparoscopic radical hysterectomy. These procedures lasted $8\frac{1}{2}$, seven and six hours respectively. These reports document the feasibility of completing these technical exercises, but further clinical experience is necessary before this approach can be recommended.

Hodgkin's disease and other malignancies

Laparoscopy has been performed for staging Hodgkin's disease for nearly 25 years but has been limited to the evaluation of hepatic and splenic involvement[25–28]. More recently there have been attempts to do complete laparoscopic staging for this disease to include pelvic and para-aortic lymph node sampling as well as splenectomy[29]. There are sure to be more reports in the future, but the adequacy of the laparoscopic staging may need to be confirmed by celiotomy before this procedure can be accepted.

As stated earlier, one of the first reports of laparoscopic evaluation of lymph nodes was by Meyer-Burg and Ziegler[7]. Their seminal report regarding gastric lymph nodes established the basis for sampling nodes associated with gastrointestinal malignancies. More recently laparoscopy has undergone comparisons with ultrasound and CT in the diagnosis of cancers of the esophagus and

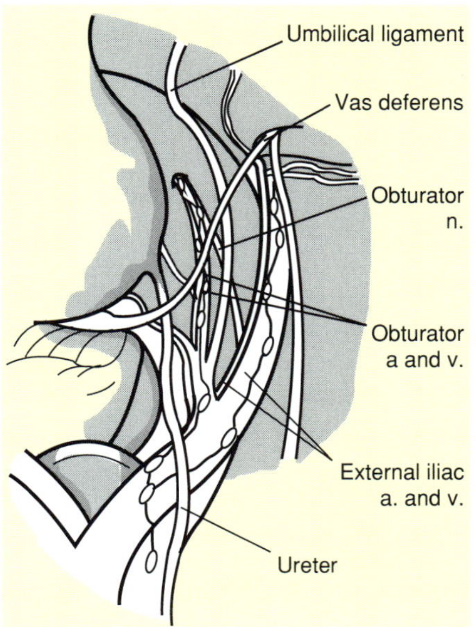

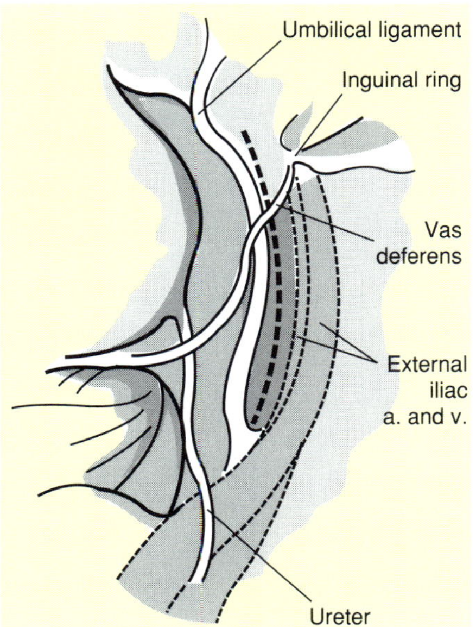

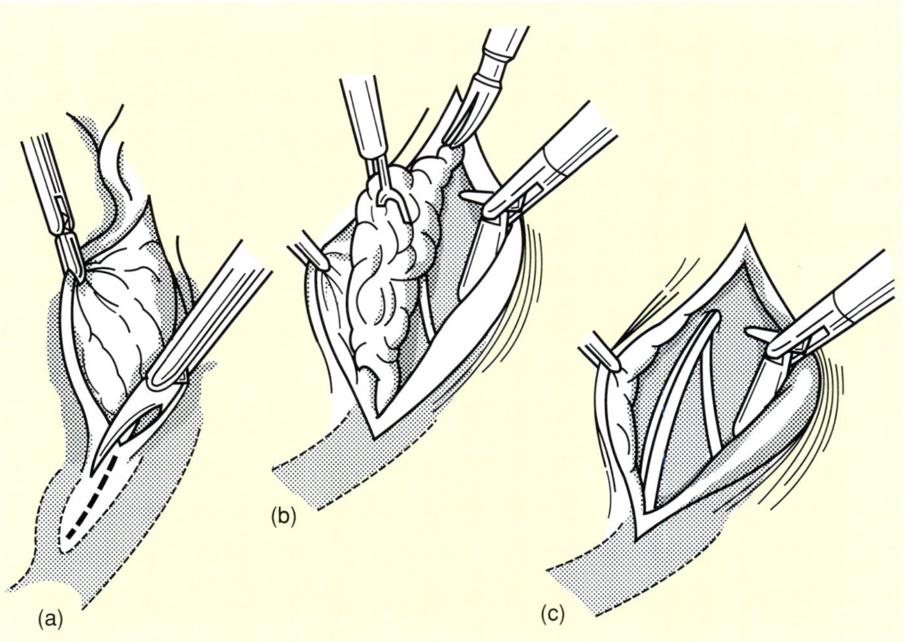

Figures 5.6–8: (Top left) Anatomy of the male pelvis. (Reprinted from Griffith *et al.*[19], by permission.) (Top right) Placement of peritoneal incision (*broken line*). (Reprinted from Griffith *et al.*[19], by permission.) Dissection of obturator lymph nodes. Lymphovascular pedicles optimally are identified before cutting to allow placement of clips, ties or electrocautery. (Reprinted from Griffith *et al.*[19], by permission.)

gastric cardia[30]. Laparoscopy was found to be significantly more sensitive and more accurate than either ultrasound or CT with regard to the detection of hepatic metastases. Laparoscopy also performed best with regard to nodal status and was the only modality to identify peritoneal metastases.

Conclusions

It is clear that laparoscopic lymph node evaluation represents a viable and potentially important modality to assess gastrointestinal malignancies, lymphomas and extra-abdominal metastases to the retroperitoneal lymph nodes. The information gained from laparoscopy may direct therapy not only by avoiding celiotomy but also to identify patients who may benefit from adjuvant therapy before surgery. A potential unexplored issue is the 'second-look' laparoscopic evaluation of lymph nodes after systemic therapy. Whatever the indication, laparoscopy is becoming an important tool in the armamentarium of the surgical oncologist.

References

1   Haagensen CD (1972) *The Lymphatics in Cancer*. W.B. Saunders, Philadelphia. pp. ix–x.

2   Kinmouth JB (1952) Lymphangiography in man. A method of outline lymphatic trunks at operation. *Clin Sci*. **11**: 13–20.

3   Kinmouth JB (1954) Lymphangiography in clinical surgery and particularly in the treatment of lymphedema. *Ann R Coll Surg*. **14**: 300–15.

4   de Roo T (1975) *Atlas of Lymphography*, Philadelphia, J.B. Lippincott. pp. 19–36.

5   Katsura Y *et al*. (1992) Endorectal ultrasonography for the assessment of wall invasion and lymph node metastasis in rectal cancer. *Dis Col Rect*. **35**: 362–8.

6   Schlag P *et al*. (1989) Scar or recurrent rectal cancer. Positron emission tomography is more helpful for diagnosis than immunoscintigraphy. *Arch Surg*. **124**: 197–200.

7   Meyer-Burg J and Ziegler U (1978) The intra-abdominal inspection and biopsy of lymph nodes during peritoneoscopy. *Endosc*. **10**: 41–3.

8   Kalk HE and Wildhirt E (1962) Lehrbuch unter Atlas der Laparoskopie und Leberpunktion. Thieme, Stuttgart.

9   Beck K (1968) Atlas der Laparoskopie. Schattaner, Stuttgart.

10   Salky BA *et al.* (1988) The use of laparoscopy in retroperitoneal pathology. *Gastrointest Endosc.* **34**: 227–30.

11   Stellato TA (1992) History of laparoscopic surgery. *Surg Clin N Am.* **72**: 997–1002.

12   Dargent D and Salvat J (1988) *Enhavissement Ganglionnaire Pelvian.* McGraw Hill, Paris. pp. 19–36.

13   Taillandier J *et al.* (1992) Pelvic lymphadenoscopy. A simple reliable method for the staging of pelvic cancer. *Internat Surg.* **77**: 211–13.

14   Ferzli G *et al.* (1992) Extraperitoneal endoscopic pelvic lymph node dissection versus laparoscopic node dissection in the staging of prostate and bladder carcinoma. *J Laparoendosc Surg.* **2**: 219–22.

15   Reich H *et al.* (1990) Laparoscopic management of stage 1 ovarian cancer. A case report. *J Reprod Med.* **35**: 601–5.

16   Querlau D *et al.* (1991) Laparoscopic pelvic lymphadenectomy in the staging of early carcinoma of the cervix. *Am J Obs Gyn.* **164**: 579–81.

17   Childers JM *et al.* (1992) The role of laparoscopic lymphadenectomy in the management of cervical carcinomas. *Gyn Oncol.* **47**: 38–43.

18   Schuessler WW *et al.* (1991) Transperitoneal endosurgical lymphadenectomy in patients with localized prostate cancer. *J Urol.* **145**: 988–91.

19   Griffith DP *et al.* (1992) Laparoscopic pelvic lymphadenectomy for prostatic adenocarcinoma. *Urol Clin N Am.* **19**: 407–15.

20   Parra RO *et al.* (1992) Staging laparoscopic pelvic lymph node dissection: comparison of results with open pelvic lymphadenectomy. *J Urol.* **147**: 875–8.

21   Harrison SH *et al.* (1992). Correlation between side of palpable tumor and side of pelvic lymph node metastasis in clinically localized prostate cancer. *Cancer.* **69**: 750–4.

22   Kavoussi LR *et al.* (1993) Complications of laparoscopic pelvic lymph node dissection. *J Urol.* **149**: 322–5.

23   Nezhat CR *et al.* (1992) Laparoscopic radical hysterectomy with paraaortic and pelvic node dissection. *Am J Obs Gyn.* **166**: 864–5.

24   Rukstalis DB *et al.* (1992) Laparoscopic retroperitoneal lymph node dissection in a patient with stage 1 testicular cancer. *J Urol.* **148**: 1907–10.

25   DeVita VT *et al.* (1971) Peritoneoscopy in the staging of Hodgkin's disease. *Canc Res.* **31**: 1746–50.

26   Beretta G *et al.* (1976) Sequential laparoscopy and laparotomy combined with bone marrow biopsy in staging Hodgkin's disease. *Canc Treat Rep.* **60**: 1231–7.

27   Chabner BA *et al.* (1976) Sequential nonsurgical and surgical staging of non-Hodgkin's lymphoma. *Ann Intern Med.* **85**: 149–54.

28   Coleman M *et al.* (1976) Peritoneoscopy in Hodgkin's disease. Confirmation of results of laparotomy. *JAMA.* **236**: 2634–6.

29   Childers JM *et al.* (1993) Laparoscopic staging of Hodgkin's Lymphoma. *J Laparoendosc Surg.* **3**: 495–7.

30   Watt I *et al.* (1989) Laparoscopy, ultrasound and computed tomography in cancers of the esophagus and gastric cardia: a prospective comparison for detecting intra-abdominal metastases. *Br J Surg.* **76**: 1036–9.

6

Laparoscopic biliary and gastric bypass

R DAVID ROSIN and SIMON PATERSON-BROWN

Introduction

When biliary and gastric bypass surgery is needed, it is almost always for patients with malignant obstruction of the distal common bile duct. The incidence of pancreatic and periampullary cancer is increasing. Over the last 50 years the increase has been twofold in Europe and the USA, threefold in Asia and fourfold in Japan. In England and Wales in 1979 the number of deaths from pancreatic cancer was 5 720. In the USA the rate per head of population was similar, ie 12.8 per 100 000 males and 11.2 per 100 000 females. 75% of all patients were more than 60 years of age and 50% were more than 70 years old. Taking account of all deaths from cancers in the USA, pancreatic cancer ranks fourth. The five-year survival rate is 2% or less, and more than 24 000 deaths are recorded annually.

Malignant obstruction of the biliary tree is amenable to curative resection in less than 10% of patients[1], and of these only 10% are alive two years later[2]. With its high incidence, poor outlook and late presentation, it is not surprising that treatment is largely palliative. Surgical palliation has an advantage on a long-term basis and offers the possibility of a single, permanent and definitive procedure[3,4]. Surgery also gives the physician a greater chance of obtaining tissue for definitive histology, allows him to confirm unresectability and provides a bypass for gastric outflow obstruction, while also affording the chance to address the problem of intractable pain, all at one time[5].

The management of patients with malignant obstruction of the distal common bile duct has undergone great changes over the last decade or so following the introduction and refinement of endoscopic techniques. The insertion of an endoprosthesis using endoscopic or percutaneous methods has provided good relief of symptoms in patients who, in addition to presenting with the biochemical and hematological sequelae of obstructed biliary flow, are often old, frail and undernourished. However, these endoscopic and percutaneous techniques may prove unsuccessful in some patients for a variety of reasons: size of tumor, anatomical abnormalities of previous surgery and duodenal obstruction, and therefore surgical intervention is required.

Furthermore, the endoprosthesis has a limited life-expectancy and may require changing more than once. The ability to perform surgical bypass using laparoscopic techniques has added a new dimension to the management of malignant obstructive jaundice, providing an alternative modality for the treatment of those patients where less invasive methods have failed. Not only can satisfactory biliary-enteric drainage be accomplished: if necessary, duodenal obstruction can also be alleviated.

There remains some controversy over which surgical bypass procedure is most appropriate for distal common bile-duct obstruction. Although several studies have failed to show statistical differences between choledocho-duodenostomy, choledocho-jejunostomy and cholecyst-jejunostomy, choledocho-jejunostomy with Roux-en-Y is the most attractive procedure on the theoretical grounds of a lower incidence of recurrent obstruction. In patients who are unwell and whose life-expectancy is very short, however, the quicker cholecyst-jejunostomy is a good alternative, provided that the cystic duct enters the common bile duct well proximal to the tumor. This chapter deals with laparoscopic cholecyst-jejunostomy, and also includes gastro-jejunostomy for those patients who also have obstruction or impending obstruction to gastric outflow.

Special diagnostic studies

Significant technical advances had been achieved thanks to improved imaging of the hepato-biliary and pancreatic ducts and parenchyma by ultrasonography, computerized axial tomography, endoscopic retrograde cholangio-pancreatography (ERCP), percutaneous transhepatic cholangiography, angiography and most recently magnetic resonance imaging and endoscopic ultrasonography.

ERCP is probably the most important of these investigations as the site of biliary and/or pancreatic obstruction is precisely defined, and the radiological pattern enables a diagnosis to be made with a higher degree of certainty. It is also helpful for demonstrating the position of entry of the cystic duct into the common hepatic duct. If ERCP fails, percutaneous transhepatic cholangiography should be performed to image the extrabiliary system.

Patient selection and preparation

Laparoscopic cholecyst-jejunostomy should be considered in patients with irresectable malignant obstruction of the lower common bile duct in whom:

- endoscopic/percutaneous stenting has failed

- the cystic duct enters the hepatic duct proximal to the tumor

- life-expectancy is 'short'. Although this is difficult to assess with confidence, a reasonable estimate can be made according to age and general condition. Patients who might live for several months should be considered for open surgical bypass using a Roux-en-Y choledocho-jejunostomy.

The patient is prepared as for open bypass surgery with adequate fluid and electrolyte resuscitation, correction of clotting abnormalities and careful monitoring of renal function. We routinely prescribe intramuscular vitamin K 10 mg daily for three days before surgery and insert a urinary catheter the day before surgery in order to maintain a urinary volume of 40–50 ml per hour with the administration of intravenous crystalloid solution.

In the operating theatre, the patient is placed on a table with facilities for X-ray or fluoroscopy and the abdomen is prepared widely as if for laparotomy. Consent is always obtained for the latter.

Surgical techniques

Initial laparoscopic assessment

After obtaining an adequate pneumoperitoneum and laparoscopic examination of the peritoneal cavity, the diagnosis is confirmed and the suitability for laparoscopic bypass assessed. This may involve the insertion of additional ports and even laparoscopic ultrasonography. Following this initial assessment, operative cholecystography is undertaken.

A spinal needle is inserted directly into the gallbladder (which is distended and must be aspirated) and contrast material is then infused. It is important to visualize free flow of contrast into the proximal biliary tree, demonstrating a patent cystic duct, and also to identify the point of insertion of the cystic duct into the common hepatic duct.

Laparoscopic cholecyst-jejunostomy

Once the decision has been made to proceed to laparoscopic bypass, the ports are inserted as shown in Figure 6.1. The duodeno-jejunal flexure (DJF) is then identified by 'walking up' the proximal jejunum using two bowel-holding (Babcock) forceps. The first loop of proximal jejunum is then brought across to the right upper quadrant in preparation for anastomosis. A small incision is then made in the fundus of the gallbladder and any residual bile removed by suction. A similar incision is then made in the jejunum. Using bowel-holding forceps, the two incisions are approximated and a linear stapler is inserted into both from the right hand side of the patient (Figure 6.2). The jejunal loop should run from the DJF directly towards the gallbladder and the lower limb of the linear stapler inserted from the distal to proximal side.

Once both limbs of the stapler have been satisfactorily inserted into each lumen, the stapling and cutting mechanisms are fired while at the same time maintaining traction on both jejunum and gallbladder to ensure that the

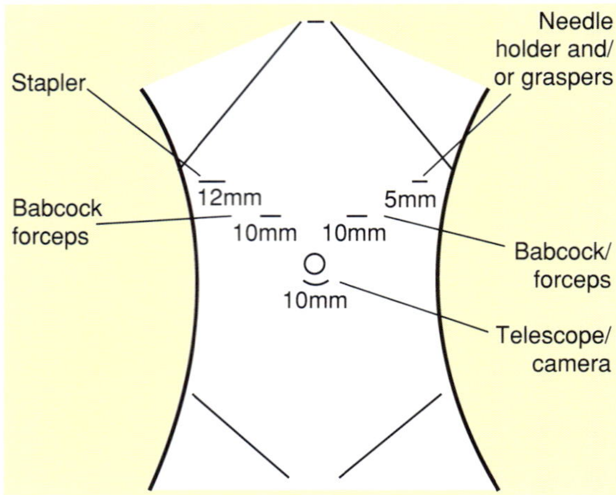

Figure 6.1: Laparoscopic cholecyst-jejunostomy: abdominal port sites.

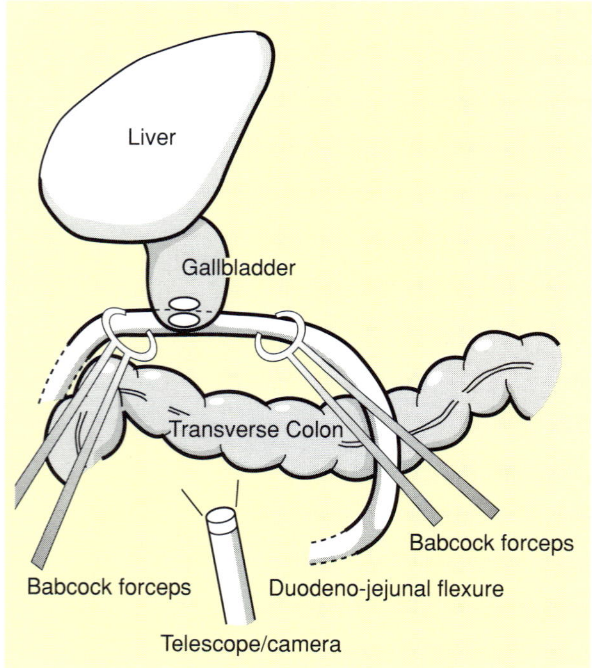

Figure 6.2: Cholecyst-jejunostomy using a linear stapler.

maximum length of wall is incorporated into the anastomosis. When the stapler is removed, the biliary enteric anastomosis will be easily seen. The anterior defect between jejunum and gallbladder where the limbs of the stapler were inserted is now closed longitudinally. This can be done using a continuous running suture or with interrupted tissue staples (Figure 6.3), such as might be used to close the peritoneum after a laparoscopic hernia repair.

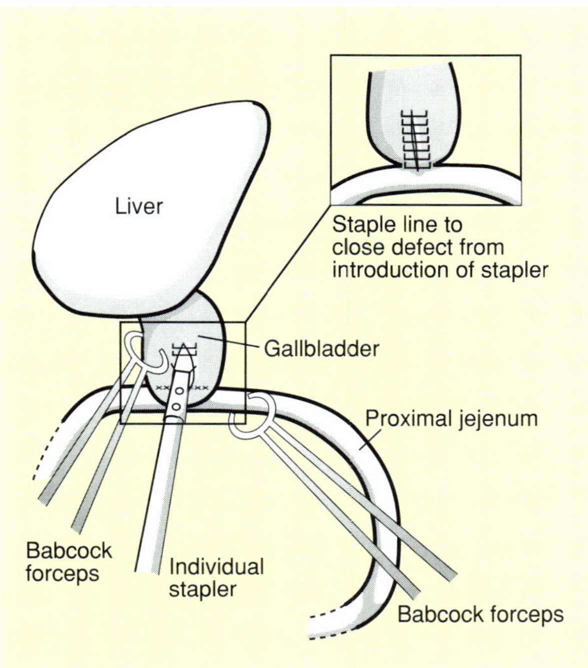

Figure 6.3: Closure of the defect made by insertion of the linear stapler using interrupted tissue staples.

Laparoscopic gastro-jejunostomy

If duodenal bypass is required, it is best done before the cholecyst-jejunostomy using the first loop of jejunum before it reaches the gallbladder. The principles are the same as for the biliary bypass. Two small incisions are made, one in the anterior surface of the antrum of the stomach, and the other in the proximal jejunum. The linear stapler is then inserted through both incisions and fired, while maintaining traction or both stomach and jejunum as shown in Figure 6.4. The defect left by the two earlier incisions expands greatly after the stapler has been fired, and owing to the thicker nature of the gastric wall, closure is best performed using sutures as opposed to staples. An inner continuous suture with outer interrupted sutures to bury the internal layer is appropriate. In some instances, it may be possible to close this defect using a linear stapler. However, care must be taken not to narrow the lumen.

Postoperative care

A nasogastric tube is left in situ after the procedure and remains until adequate gastric emptying has been established. Then it is removed and oral diet is commenced according to the patient's clinical condition. The authors give three doses of parenteral antibiotic chemo-prophylaxis in the perioperative period, but thereafter patient condition dictates management.

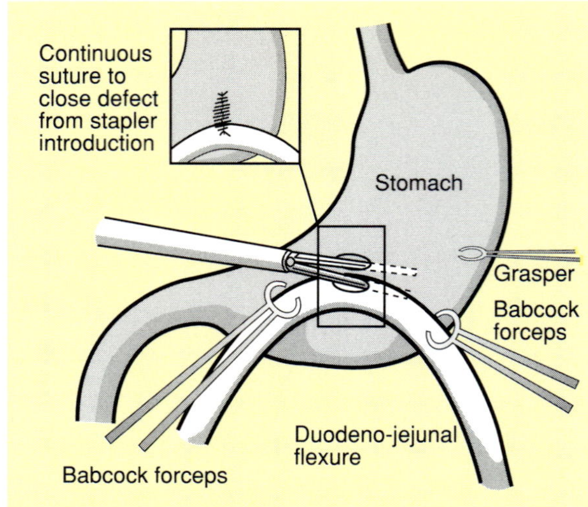

Figure 6.4: Insertion of the linear stapler when forming the gastro-jejunostomy.

Discussion

In a selected group of patients, laparoscopic biliary-enteric bypass has a role to play and extends the treatment options available for the palliation of malignant obstructive jaundice of the distal common bile duct. It remains to be seen whether there are patients who might benefit from laparoscopic cholecyst-jejunostomy more than from endoscopic stenting, with regard to recurrent jaundice from blocked stents, and results from current prospective trials are eagerly awaited. At the time of writing, however, the indications for the laparoscopic procedure remain strictly limited to those patients in whom endoscopic or percutaneous stenting has failed and whose life-expectancy and general condition suggest that open surgical bypass would be inappropriate.

References

1   Koven IH *et al.* (1981) Percutaneous ante-grade biliary damage: a non-operative approach to biliary obstruction. *Can J Surg.* **24:** 591–3.

2   Huang JF and Little JM (1987) Malignant jaundice. *Aust NZ J Surg.* **57:** 505–9.

3   De Rooji PD *et al.* (1991) Evaluation of palliative surgical procedures in unresectable cancer. *Br J Surg.* **78:** 1053–8.

4   Jones RS (1991) Palliative operative procedures for carcinoma of the gall bladder. *World J Surg.* **15:** 348–51.

5   Wanatapa P and Williamson RCN (1992) Surgical palliation for pancreatic cancer: developments during the past two decades. *Br J Surg.* **79:** 8–20.

7

Laparoscopic evaluation and resection of the spleen in cancer management

EDWARD H PHILLIPS and RAUL J ROSENTHAL

Introduction

Throughout history, the spleen has excited the imagination of philosophers and physicians. There is no mention of the spleen in the Bible, but its anatomy, functions and disorders are discussed in the Babylonian Talmud[1]. Galen described it as 'misterii plenum organum', an organ full of mystery. It was believed that the spleen extracted the malancholic humors from blood and thus was associated with merriment and laughter—'great laughers have great spleens'. It was also thought to cause 'heaviness', and that is removal would allow one to run faster[2].

In 1549, Leonardo Fioravanti of Naples reported the first splenectomy. The operation was allegedly performed by Adriano Zacarello, but the veracity of this report is still a subject of debate among surgical historians[3]. Not until the 17th century did an accurate understanding of the anatomy of the spleen emerge from autopsy and animal research. Investigators such as Harvey, Glisson, Bartholin, Wharton and Virchow described the structure of the spleen in detail[4].

In 1826, Quittenbaum of Rostock performed the first undisputed splenectomy. The patient lived for only six hours. At autopsy the ligature was found intact, but the liver was small, hard and cirrhotic. This was clearly a case of secondary hypersplenism due to portal hypertension. The second authenticated (but again fatal) case was described in 1855 by Küchler of Darmastadt. The patient died two hours after surgery, because of hemorrhage from a small branch of the splenic artery. In 1865 Sir T Spencer Wells, a prominent Victorian surgeon, reported these first two cases and his own case (the third in the world literature) of splenectomy operated with the preoperative diagnosis of abdominal tumor. The patient died 158 hours after the operation. At autopsy the patient had signs of rigor suggesting septicemia[5].

Although there are references to splenectomy being performed in the early 1800s, the first documented successful splenectomy for a pathologically enlarged spleen was reported by Jules Péan in 1867. The patient was a woman of 20 who had a painful abdominal mass that was thought to be an ovarian tumor. At operation the tumor was found to be a splenic cyst. The spleen was removed and the patient recovered[6].

In 1888 Wells reported the results of 52 cases from several surgical centers, and found that complete excision of the spleen had a mortality of 63%[7]. He concluded that operations performed before 1848 had a very high mortality because they were performed without anesthesia, and that operations performed before 1875 had a high mortality because they were performed without antiseptic precautions.

In 1908, in a lecture at John Hopkins Hospital, George Ben Johnston reported an improvement in the technique of splenectomy. This technique has remained essentially unchanged to the present day. From 1890 to 1908 refinements in surgical techniques decreased the mortality rate to 20%[8]. The next significant improvement in outcome after splenectomy occurred when Landsteiner discovered blood types. This led to the use of life-saving transfusions. The development of blood-banking in the early 1940s, along with improvements in general anesthesia, further improved the outcome of splenectomy[9].

As late as 1952, the spleen was considered non-essential to life. King and Shumaker[10] challenged this concept when they reported five infants who developed fulminant bacterial infection shortly after splenectomy for congenital hemolytic anemia. Subsequent research has established the immunologic role of the spleen. The spleen began to be regarded not as a disposable organ but as one that had important immunological function in children and to some extent in adults. The thought that the spleen should be preserved if possible led to the development of the technique of partial splenectomy in the 1960s[11–13].

There are still many indications for splenectomy, however especially in the management of cancer. This chapter highlights the major clinical, pathological and surgical features of splenic tumors, with specific emphasis on the surgical approach. The technique of laparoscopic splenectomy is also presented, along with its indications and contraindications.

Splenic tumors

There are several methods of categorizing splenic tumors. Morgenstern and Geller used four major categories[14]: tumor-like lesions (cystic and pseudocysts), vascular tumors, lymphoid tumors, and non-lymphoid tumors (Table 7.1).

Cystic lesions of the spleen

Splenic cysts are relatively uncommon abdominal tumors[15,16]. Two basic types of splenic cysts have been described: primary cysts (true epidermoid cysts) with cellular lining, and secondary cysts (pseudocysts) without epithelium[17]. Non-parasitic splenic cysts seem ideally suited to laparoscopic treatment[12].

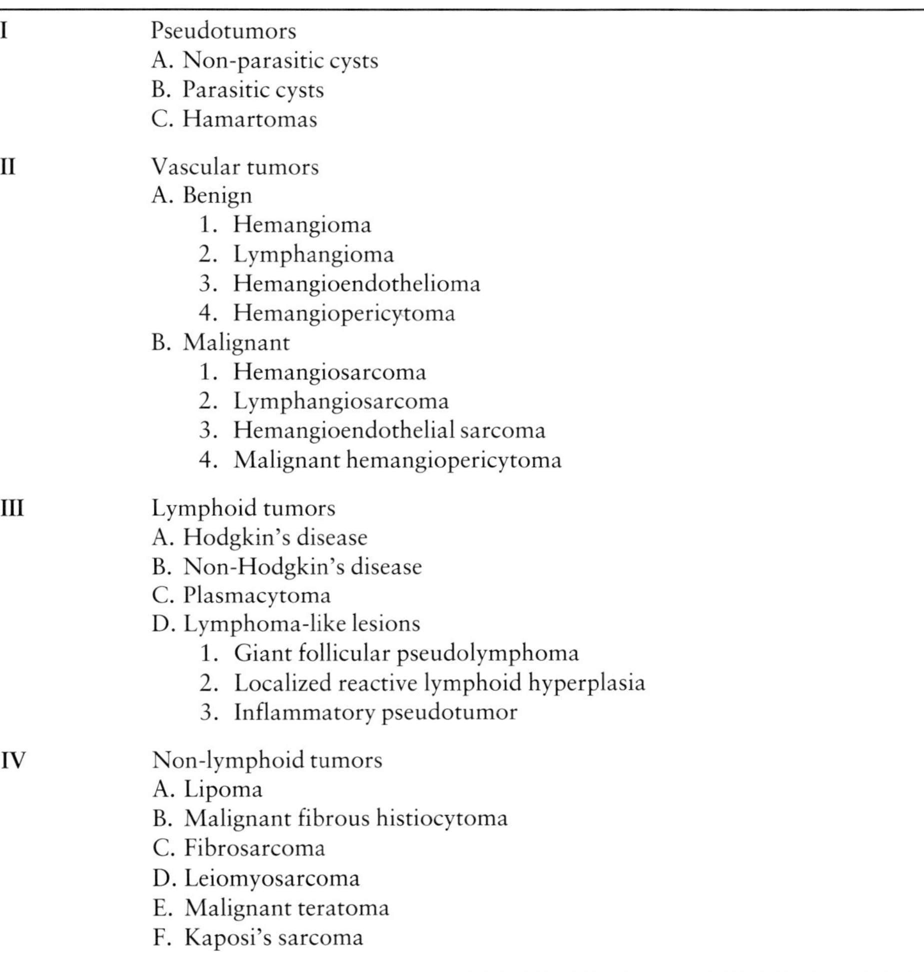

I	Pseudotumors
	A. Non-parasitic cysts
	B. Parasitic cysts
	C. Hamartomas
II	Vascular tumors
	A. Benign
	1. Hemangioma
	2. Lymphangioma
	3. Hemangioendothelioma
	4. Hemangiopericytoma
	B. Malignant
	1. Hemangiosarcoma
	2. Lymphangiosarcoma
	3. Hemangioendothelial sarcoma
	4. Malignant hemangiopericytoma
III	Lymphoid tumors
	A. Hodgkin's disease
	B. Non-Hodgkin's disease
	C. Plasmacytoma
	D. Lymphoma-like lesions
	1. Giant follicular pseudolymphoma
	2. Localized reactive lymphoid hyperplasia
	3. Inflammatory pseudotumor
IV	Non-lymphoid tumors
	A. Lipoma
	B. Malignant fibrous histiocytoma
	C. Fibrosarcoma
	D. Leiomyosarcoma
	E. Malignant teratoma
	F. Kaposi's sarcoma

Table 7.1:   Primary tumors of the spleen.

Primary splenic cysts

This group can be divided into parasitic and non-parasitic (either congenital or neoplastic) cysts. Parasitic cysts are five to 10 times as common as non-parasitic cysts, though there are no accurate data about the true incidence of non-parasitic cysts of the spleen. Garvin and King studied 102 cysts, and only two (1.9%) of them were parasitic[18]. Primary cysts have a squamous epithelial lining, although some may occasionally have a mesothelial lining (Figure 7.1). It is thought that the squamous or the mesothelial-lined cysts originate as inclusions of mesothelium which are retained in the spleen during embryogenesis. They can undergo metaplasia[19].

There is a rarer form of splenic cyst in which the squamous epithelium is keratinized. Some have suggested that these cysts may be neoplastic instead of metaplastic. In one study of ovarian epidermoid cysts, ultrastructural data supported the possible origin from metaplastic mesothelium[18].

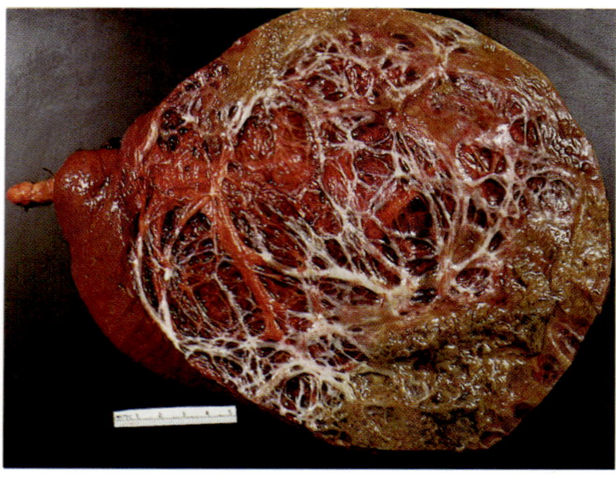

Figure 7.1: Epidermoid cyst of the spleen.

Secondary cysts

Secondary (pseudo) cysts (Figure 7.2) are more common than primary cysts. Their pathogenesis is thought to be well understood. In many cases, trauma is cited as the contributing factor. It is thought that trauma leads to intrasplenic hemorrhage. The hematoma that forms becomes encapsulated; subsequently the blood is absorbed and the false cyst wall persists. It can eventually become thick fibrous tissue with extensive calcification. The presence of radiographically visible calcification is not however a reliable feature to differentiate secondary from primary cysts, since primary cyst walls can also calcify[20].

Vascular tumors of the spleen

Hemangiomas

Vascular neoplasms or hemangiomas are the most common primary splenic tumors[21]. They are usually found at autopsy or in spleens removed for other reasons. Their rupture is uncommon. Macroscopically they usually appear as blood-filled cysts, either singly or in groups. Histologically they are most often

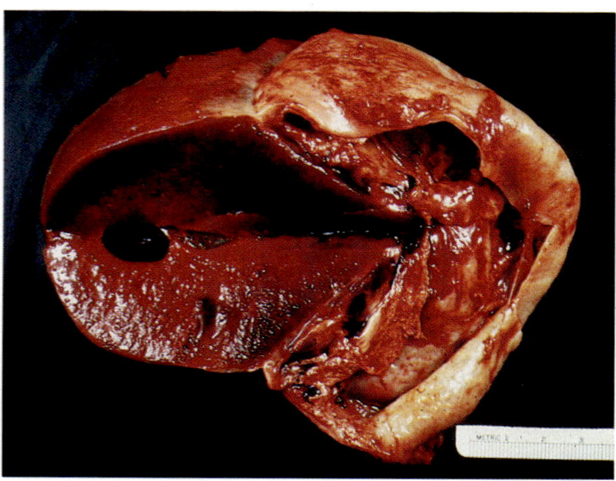

Figure 7.2: Secondary (pseudo) cyst of the spleen. Traumatic etiology.

cavernous in pattern, but capillary-type hemangiomas may be seen. The usual picture is that of vascular spaces lined by a single layer of bland endothelial cells without mitosis. They are only rarely mistaken for malignant tumors grossly.

Lymphangiomas

Lymphangiomas are multiple or single neoplasms. They consist of endothelial-lined capsular cysts filled with eosinophilic proteinaceous material. Discovery is usually accidental, although some patients with lymphangiomatous cysts may present with splenomegaly[22,23].

Angiosarcomas

Angiosarcoma or hemangiosarcoma of the spleen have been associated with environmental or work-related factors such as thorium dioxide and monomeric vinyl chloride[24]. Nevertheless, primary hemangiosarcomas of the spleen are rare. Usually the spleen is involved when hemangiosarcoma develops in other adjacent organs such as the liver.

Angiosarcoma, hemangiosarcoma and hemangioendothelialsarcoma are most likely the same tumor (Figure 7.3). Hemangiosarcoma is the preferred term, and distinguishes this tumor from lymphangiosarcoma. The neoplastic and malignant nature of the tumor is not always obvious initially. Hemangiosarcoma may present as splenomegaly, angiopathic hemolytic anemia or ascites or with spontaneous rupture[25-27]. Prognosis is invariably poor[28].

Primary non-lymphoid tumors of the spleen

Hamartomas

Hamartomas are rare, benign splenic lesions. Rokitansky was the first to report them, and termed them 'splenomas'[29]. Their incidence has been estimated to be 1.5 in 100,000. They are mostly found incidentally at autopsy. They are also occasionally palpated during abdominal surgery. They appear in patients of all ages; although they appear to be more frequent in older people, this may be a

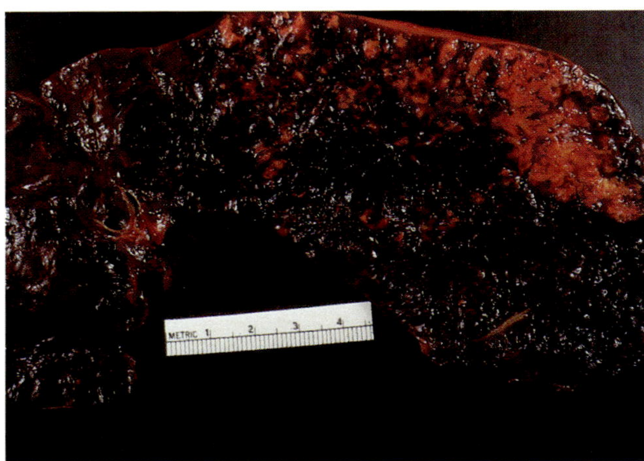

Figure 7.3: Spleen involved by hemangiosarcoma.

bias due to their usual mode of discovery. They typically appear as well circumscribed (often non-encapsulated) lesions which bulge from the cut surface, and are darker than the surrounding spleen (Figure 7.4). Microscopically the lesion is easily recognized because of the slit-like and tortuous endothelial-lined spaces and the distinct border.

With the increased reliance on imaging techniques such as computerized tomography and magnetic resonance imaging, splenomas may be discovered more frequently in the future. Differential diagnosis can be difficult. Rarely, hamartomas are multiple and distributed widely enough throughout the spleen to cause splenomegaly and hypersplenism. Short of excision, the diagnosis is impossible to make. However, if the patient is asymptomatic and a single lesion is discovered incidentally by palpation or scans, there is a role for observation.

Primary lymphoid splenic neoplasm

Although the spleen is often the site of secondary involvement by Hodgkin's disease and the non-Hodgkin's lymphomas, primary lymphoid malignancies (Figure 7.5) can occur[21,30–32]. When lymphoma does involve the spleen, either as a primary or secondary process, the white pulp is involved first. There may be diffuse involvement (in the case of nodular lymphomas) or large irregular tumor masses (as in the case of large cell lymphomas). By contrast, malignant tumors of true histiocytic origin (Figure 7.6) frequently involve the spleen diffusely and splenomegaly may be the only abnormal physical sign[33].

Other lymphoproliferative diseases may also cause splenomegaly and may mimic lymphoma. Castleman's tumor (angiofollicular lymphoid hyperplasia) occurs either as a solitary lesion or as part of a diffuse lymphoid hyperplasia syndrome[34]. Castleman's tumor is thought to be a true lymphoid hamartoma

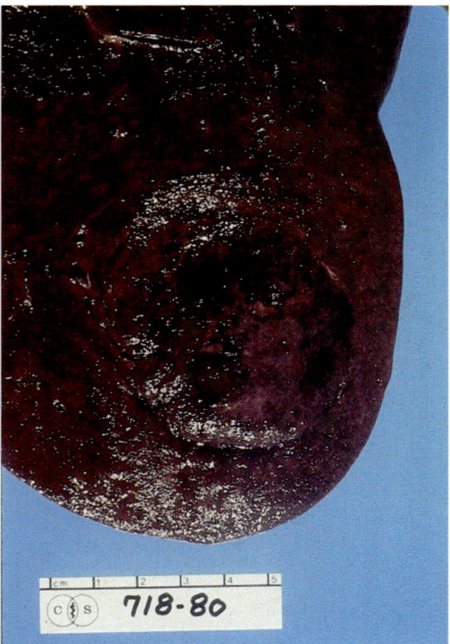

Figure 7.4:   Hamartoma of the spleen. These tumors are also termed splenomas.

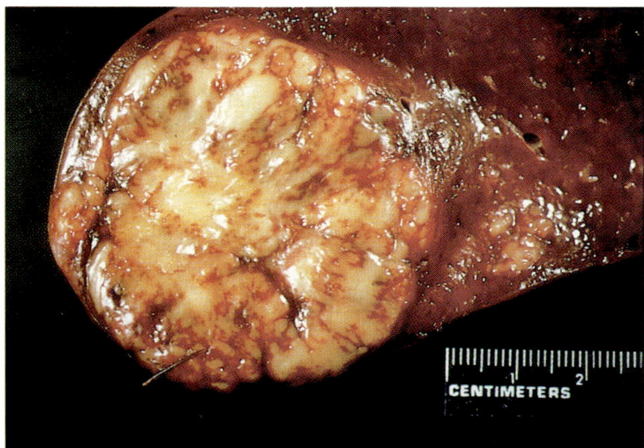

Figure 7.5: Nodular Hodgkin's disease; note multiple white tumor nodules which are confluent.

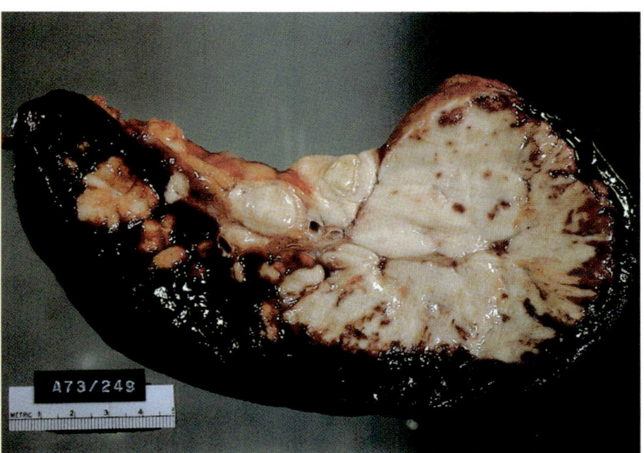

Figure 7.6: Histiocytic lymphoma of the spleen.

but does not resemble the follicular pattern of splenic hamartoma described by Berge[35]

Primary plasmacytoma (Figure 7.7) is very rare and is not grossly recognizable. This is an inflammatory cell mass which does not resemble hamartomas, but must be distinguished from lymphomas[36].

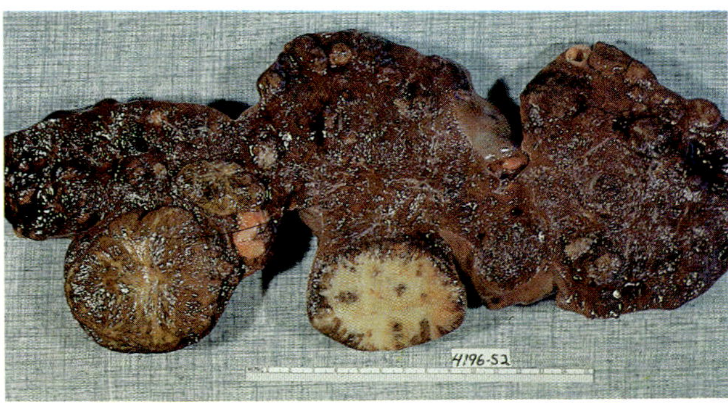

Figure 7.7: Plasmacytoma of the spleen.

Non-lymphoid tumors

Lipomas, angiomyolipomas, fibrous histiocytomas and sarcomas

Lipomas, angiomyolipomas and fibrous histiocytomas have occasionally been reported to involve the spleen[37,38]. Several cases of primary splenic malignant fibrous histiocytoma have also been described. Though they usually occur in the soft tissues, they have also been found in a number of organs including the spleen. They result in massive splenomegaly and tend to be quite aggressive. The histogenesis of these tumors remains the subject of debate[39,40].

Malignant fibrous histiocytoma may be misdiagnosed as fibrosarcoma or leiomyosarcoma, both of which occur in the spleen[30,37]. There is a single report of a malignant teratoma with papillary carcinoma, spindle cell sarcoma and cartilaginous tissue[41].

Kaposi's sarcoma

In recent years, Kaposi's sarcoma has become more common with the increasing prevalence of AIDS. Kaposi's sarcoma is a spindle cell malignant neoplasm characterized by vascular spaces not generally lined by endothelial cells. There is often extravasation of blood in the spindle cell areas and there may be a variable plasma cell component. Kaposi's sarcoma does not usually present as a primary splenic tumor. It occurs in patients in whom the spleen is involved as part of a general sarcomatosis (Figure 7.8).

Metastatic tumors involving the spleen

Metastasis to the spleen is found in only 7% of autopsied cancer patients. Melanoma, lung and breast cancer are the tumor types that most frequently metastasize to the spleen[39,42]. Nevertheless, virtually every tumor has been known to metastasize to the spleen. They may present as pain or splenomegaly or with spontaneous rupture (Figure 7.9).

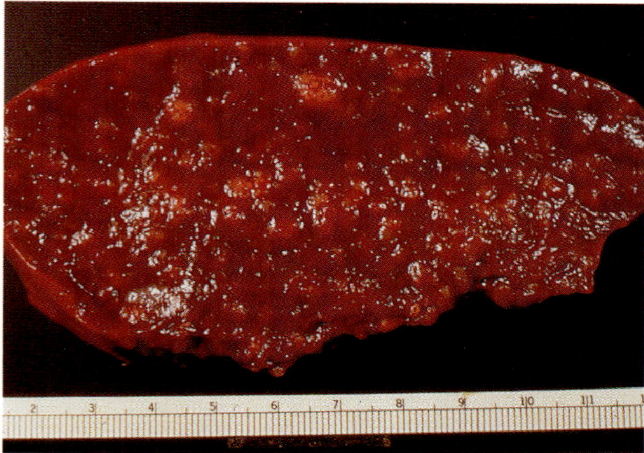

Figure 7.8: Sarcoma of the spleen.

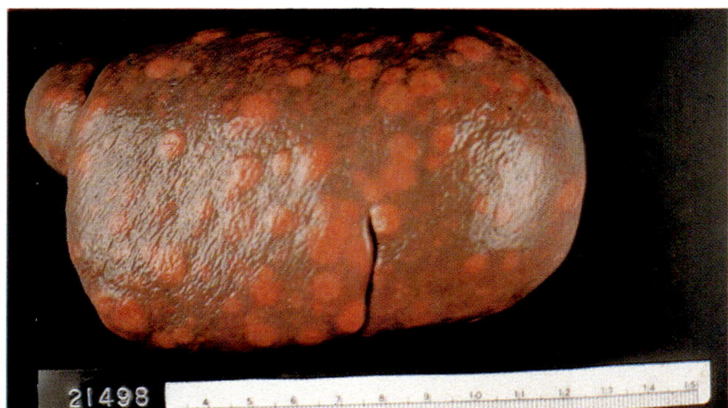

Figure 7.9: Metastasis of ovarian cancer involving the spleen.

The role of surgery in the treatment of Hodgkin's disease and other lymphomas

Throughout the 19th century, the therapy for Hodgkin's disease and other lymphomas was symptomatic and palliative. In 1902, Pusey was apparently the first to treat lymphomas with X-rays (newly discovered by Roentgen in 1896). The second report on the treatment of Hodgkin's disease with irradiation came from Chicago in 1903. Nicholas Senn, professor of surgery at Rush Medical College, described dramatic responses in two patients treated with irradiation[43]. For decades the role of surgery was to biopsy palpably involved tissue in order to document the presence of Hodgkin's disease. Between 1920 and 1950 there was some interest in the use of radical surgery for the eradication of localized lymphomas. In those series in which good results were reported, X-ray therapy had been given postoperatively. Eventually, critical review of these studies led most surgeons to believe that radical surgery was not indicated in the primary management of malignant lymphomas[42].

In the 1940s, as a by-product of wartime work on compounds related to the mustard gases, it was discovered that the nitrogen mustards had powerful lymphocytolytic effects on normal lymphoid tissues. Clinical trials in selected cases of Hodgkin's disease and other malignant lymphomas confirmed a similar response[44]. This was the beginning of chemotherapy for lymphomas and leukemias, helped later in the same decade by the development of other chemotherapeutic agents.

In 1958, Peters[45] demonstrated that the extent of the disease correlated with survival in patients treated with radiation therapy. The 10-year survival rates were established as 58%, 35% and 2% for stages I, II and III respectively. This laid the groundwork for the present system of staging the extent of disease (see Chapter 4).

Improved survival rates in clinical stage I–II Hodgkin's disease were achieved during the 1960s with extended field irradiation and adjuvant chemotherapy[46–48]. In 1964, experimental studies showed the desirability of using combinations of agents with non-overlapping toxicities. This led to the introduction of the highly effective MOPP (mustard, oncovin, procarbazine, prednisone) regimen[49]. Chemotherapy has become the primary treatment for patients with stage IV and stage III B disease, while those with stage I, II, and III A are treated with irradiation.

In 1969, the group at Stanford University[50] recommended a new surgical procedure for staging of Hodgkin's disease: laparotomy with splenectomy, liver biopsy and biopsy of lymph nodes in various locations. This approach yielded a high incidence of occult disease in patients with no other clinical or radiological evidence of infradiaphragmatic involvement[51].

Fabri *et al.*[52] reported in 1974 that staging laparotomy for Hodgkin's disease altered the staging in about half of 77 cases. 12% were down-staged and in 38% the staging was higher. Mortality was 0%. During the same period, Cannon *et al.*[53] published similar results. Major morbidity was 4% and mortality was 0%, though only 28% had their clinical staging changed. Ferguson *et al.*[54] reported on 125 patients who underwent staging laparotomy for lymphoma. They experienced one death and a morbidity of 5%. 25% were under-staged and 27% were over-staged. Ferguson showed that 21% of macroscopic normal-looking spleens were histologically pathologic.

Nevertheless improvements in diagnostic radiology, concomitant with improvements in chemotherapy and radiation therapy, led investigators to question the routine use of staging laparotomy[55]. The European Organization for Research and Treatment of Cancer showed that there was no significant difference in survival between patients who had staging laparotomies and those who did not, as long as recurrences were treated with 'salvage' chemotherapy[56].

If it is concluded that staging laparotomy provides no survival benefit, why stage patients? It is certainly important to down-stage patients and avoid unnecessary treatment and its complications. 6% of patients treated with radiation and chemotherapy will get leukemia and/or lymphomas on average seven and 20 years later, respectively. Additionally, 10 to 12% of treated patients will get second tumors such as melanoma, breast cancer and sarcoma[57].

Chemotherapy in a salvage situation also increases morbidity because the patients have previously undergone radiation therapy which has limited their bone marrow capacity. Properly staging patients initially affords one treatment that avoids the radiation therapy and its effects in stage III and IV patients. Additionally, staging laparotomy in young female patients affords an opportunity to perform oophoropexies, thus protecting the ovaries if subsequent radiation of the pelvic lymph nodes is required[58].

There are reports that certain cell types confined to high cervical lymph nodes have less chance of infradiaphragmatic involvement and mixed cellularity, and nodular sclerosing tumor types also have less incidence of stage III and IV disease. However, staging laparotomy should not be denied to individual patients on that basis, though there is some controversy on this point. Before recommending a staging laparotomy, the patient's overall medical condition and age should be considered because it is a formidable operation. Still, it has a remarkably low morbidity (10–25%) and mortality rates (0–5%)[59–63]. This is probably because most patients are young (average age 40 years) and otherwise healthy.

In 1992, Musser *et al.*[64] reported the UCLA experience with 306 patients who underwent laparotomy and splenectomy for hematologic diseases. In 40 cases, splenectomy was performed for staging in Hodgkin's disease with a morbidity of 10% and a mortality of 5%. The mortality rate should be below 1% if it is to be recommended to patients who have no evidence of infradiaphragmatic disease. It is hoped that laparoscopic staging will provide useful information with minimal morbidity and mortality.

Restaging laparotomy is occasionally necessary to exclude recurrence or the emergence of non-Hodgkin's lymphoma[65]. Laparoscopy is more difficult in the previously operated abdomen but offers a minimal access approach to specific enlarged lymph nodes or liver nodules.

Staging for non-Hodgkin's lymphoma

Routine staging for non-Hodgkin's lymphoma remains controversial and is not widely practiced. More often splenectomy or liver biopsy is required to diagnose recurrences or second tumors. Laparoscopy with directed liver biopsy and/or laparoscopic splenectomy is useful in this setting. Recently we performed a laparoscopic splenectomy in a 64-year-old male who developed several 1 cm nodules in his spleen three years after chemotherapy for mixed and diffuse lymphoma found in a cervical lymph node. Pathologic analysis confirmed a recurrence of his original cell type.

Splenectomy in patients with advanced Hodgkin's disease, non-Hodgkin's lymphoma, or leukemia complicated by hemolytic anemia, pancytopenia and hypersplenism

The excellent surgical results seen with splenectomy in patients with Hodgkin's disease are distinctly different from the results when splenectomy is performed in the face of hypersplenism. When advanced Hodgkin's disease or lymphoma is complicated by hemolytic anemia, thrombocytopenia and/or leukopenia, morbidity and mortality is higher than when performed electively for staging[66,67]. Neal *et al.*[68] reported on 50 patients who were treated with splenectomy for advanced chronic lymphocytic leukemia. A positive response was achieved in 77% of patients with hemolytic anemia, 70% of patients with thrombocytopenia and 64% of patients with both anemia and thrombocytopenia. 80% of responders continued to exhibit a good response at one year. Postoperative transfusion requirements decreased in responders. However, the operative morbidity was 26% and the operative mortality was 4%. The mean duration of hospitalization was 9.8 days.

Delpero *et al.*[69] published their experience with 62 patients who underwent splenectomy for hypersplenism due to chronic lymphocytic leukemia or non-Hodgkin's lymphoma. All had splenomegaly and half had massive splenomegaly. Forty nine had thrombocytopenia, 16 had anemia, six had leukopenia, 15 had anemia with thrombocytopenia and three had pancytopenia. There was a 29% morbidity rate and a 1.6% mortality rate. 89% responded in the first month but only 63% had a response at two years. Bone marrow depletion did not preclude a response to splenectomy.

Splenectomy in the treatment of hairy-cell leukemia

Damasio *et al.*[70] published preliminary results of a multi-center study in Italy that included 115 patients. They studied the effects of splenectomy after induction therapy with alpha interferon. The treatment groups were randomized to splenectomy or observation if they responded to 12 months of interferon therapy. Thirteen patients were randomized and splenectomy was performed in only six patients. Splenectomy prolonged the response to interferon therapy in comparison to controls in this continuing study.

Musser and colleagues at UCLA[64] reported ten cases of splenectomy for hairy cell leukemia and found a response in five cases, with 19% morbidity and 6% mortality. However, the role of splenectomy is being reevaluated because of recent successes with infusion chemotherapy with 2-chlorodeoxy-adenosine. Piro *et al.*[71] have reported a roughly 80% durable remission rate following a single course of treatment with this drug.

Splenectomy in the treatment of gastric, pancreatic and colon cancer

Hopes that adding splenectomy to radical gastrectomy for cure of gastric malignancy would increase survival rates have not been realized. Maehara *et al.*[72] and Brady *et al.*[73] have published large series of patients studied retrospectively, showing that adding splenectomy to partial or total gastrectomy for cure increases morbidity and mortality while not improving survival rates.

Likewise, the addition of incidental splenectomy to pancreatic and colon resections for malignancy significantly increases morbidity and mortality without increasing survival. Fabri *et al.*[52] found a 44% morbidity and a 14% mortality compared to a 32% morbidity and a 5% mortality without splenectomy.

Splenectomy in the treatment of ovarian cancer

Splenectomy appears justified in rare cases when the spleen is involved with epithelial ovarian cancer and splenectomy is performed in conjunction with cytoreductive surgery in preparation for intensive chemotherapy. Sonnendecker and colleagues[74] reported on six such cases (Figure 7.9). One patient had diffuse parenchymal involvement. Three patients were alive with no evidence of disease with as long as a 32-month follow-up. One patient died of a pulmonary embolus postoperatively.

Clinical features of splenic tumors

No constant clinical symptom or sign can be attributed to this group of such diverse pathologic conditions of the spleen. Nevertheless, the most common clinical finding is splenomegaly. Splenomegaly is usually discovered because of complaints of left upper abdominal discomfort or pain. Massively enlarged spleens displace and compress adjacent organs. Symptoms such as postprandial satiety, dyspnea, shoulder pain and even constipation can be present.

If the lesion is localized to only a portion of the spleen, no hematological changes may be present. If the process is diffuse, the phenomena of sequestration may be manifested by anemia, granulocytopenia and/or thrombocytopenia. Systemic signs such as fever, pleural effusion and cachexia should lead one to suspect a malignant process though repeated splenic infarcts can mimic malignancy. Splenic infarcts can also cause pleuritic pain and fever. Finally, splenic neoplasms may rupture spontaneously or as the result of minimal trauma causing an acute abdomen[14].

Surgical considerations of splenectomy and preoperative splenic artery embolization

Conventional splenectomy by laparotomy has evolved from decades of surgical experience. It has become an operation performed by every community general surgeon with acceptable morbidity and mortality in elective cases. The rapid development of advanced minimal access surgical techniques has led inevitably to the development of laparoscopic techniques of splenectomy. The advantages of minimal access procedures are decreased postoperative discomfort, shorter hospital stays, and earlier resumption of normal activities[75-78]. The evidence that morbidity and mortality is reduced in advanced laparoscopic procedures is emerging but hardly proven[79]. The results in laparoscopic splenectomy are no exception to this experience.

The main indications for laparoscopic splenectomy are diseases in which the spleen is normal or minimally enlarged, such as idiopathic thrombocytopenic purpura (sometimes related to AIDS), and/or hemolytic anemias. In the case of splenic tumors, it is important to distinguish between benign and malignant diseases. Benign tumors can be operated on totally laparoscopically. Malignant ones are often associated with significant splenomegaly and require incisions for specimen removal and careful technique for tumor cell isolation. Staging operations for Hodgkin's disease are ideal cases as the spleen is usually of normal size and the patients are relatively young and healthy. A counterincision is required to remove the splenic specimen and lymph node specimens for pathologic analysis.

If the spleen/tumor is enlarged, the patient's body habitus becomes the determining factor in allowing adequate exposure of the splenic hilum.

Preoperative splenic artery embolization is helpful in reducing the size of the spleen and decreasing operative time in these borderline cases. Indications are:

- splenomegaly

- relative inexperience of the surgeon

- obesity

- prior upper abdominal surgery

- AIDS.

Good exposure is critical. Accurate dissection and hemostasis is vital. Visualization is aided by the magnification of the laparoscope but technique and operative sequencing are critical to the safe and successful outcome of splenectomy.

Technique

Patients should receive preoperative immunization with a pneumococcal vaccine such as Pneumovax, and possibly also with hemophilus influenza and meningococcus vaccines. Autologous blood is obtained for all elective cases. Operations are performed under general anesthesia. Preoperative splenic artery embolization is considered in obese patients or patients with splenomegaly. Patients are positioned on a beanbag on an electric operating table for easier position change during surgery. This becomes an important issue during a laparoscopic splenectomy, especially when dissecting the splenorenal and the splenophrenic ligaments. A 30⊃ viewing-angled laparoscope is preferred.

Following creation of the pneumoperitoneum with a Verres needle or open technique, a 10/11 mm trocar is placed in the umbilical area and a general inspection of the abdomen is performed. A 5 or 10/11 mm trocar is placed in the subxiphoid area, and a 10/11 mm trocar (the operating trocar) is placed halfway between the subxiphoid and the umbilical trocar. A 10/11 mm trocar (the lateral trocar) is placed in the left axillary line, halfway between the costal margin and the iliac crest. A 12 mm trocar (the stapler trocar) is placed halfway between the umbilicus and the lateral trocar.

The operation is begun by ligating the splenic artery in the lesser sac. (Figure 7.10 **a, b**). The stomach is reflected anteriorly, and the colon retracted inferiorly with Babcock graspers placed via the two lateral trocars. A window in the gastrocolic omentum is opened with scissors or electrocautery. The pancreas is retracted posteriorly and inferiorly with a fan retractor. The tortuous splenic artery is usually pushed up into view by this maneuver. The peritoneum overlying the artery is lifted with a grasper placed via the subxiphoid trocar and divided by a scissors placed via the operating trocar. The splenic artery is then grasped, elevated and occluded with a large endoclip (Figure 7.10 **c**).

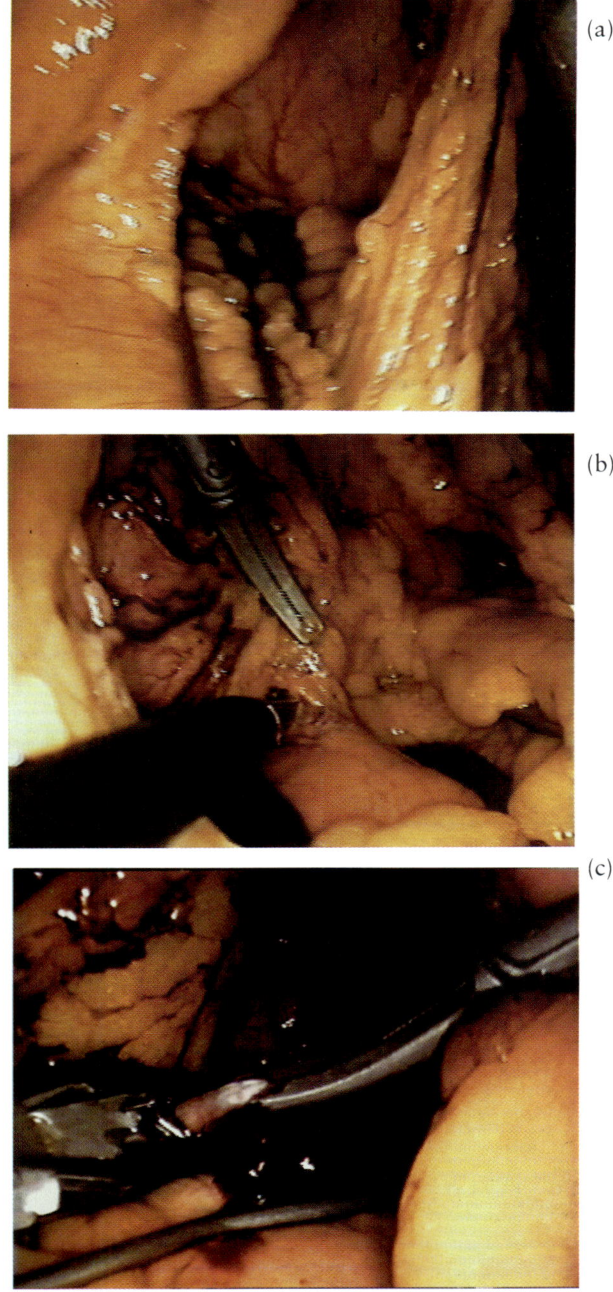

Figure 7.10: Occlusion of the splenic artery. (a) view into the lesser sac, (b) dissection of the artery, (c) occlusion of the splenic artery with a clip.

Attention is then paid to the colosplenic attachments. They are divided sharply or with a hook or right angle tipped electrocautery. (Figure 7.11). The spleen is then grasped with a ring forceps grasper and elevated anteriorly and medially via the lateral trocar (with the patient positioned left side up). The splenorenal ligament is divided with scissors and/or electrocautery hook. An electrocautery hook device with suction and irrigation facilitates this maneuver

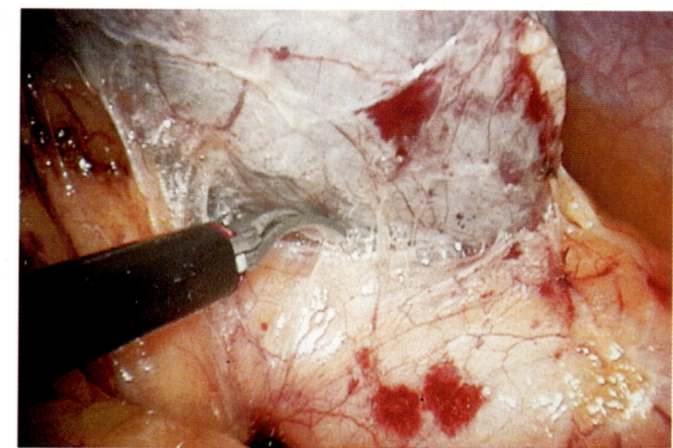

(a)

(b)

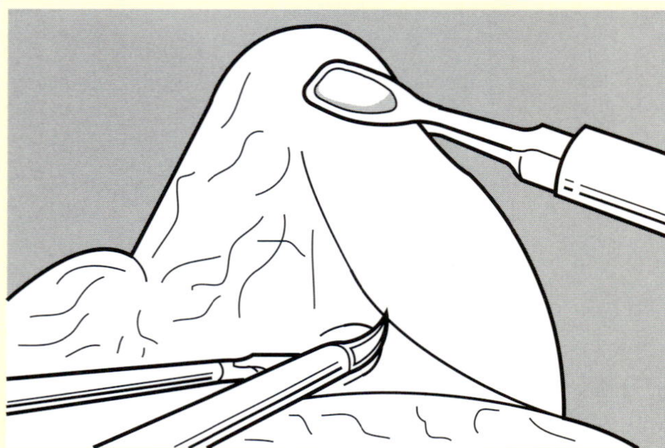

Figure 7.11:   Dissection of colosplenic attachments.

and increases visualization. The dissection is taken cephalad as far as possible. Division of the splenophrenic attachments allows the spleen to be completely elevated, exposing the hilar vessels. If splenomegaly prevents extensive mobilization, the operation is more difficult and more dangerous. The inferior hilar vessels are divided until more of the retrosplenic splenorenal and or splenophrenic attachments can be divided. Though some advocate dividing the hilar vessels first[80–82], bleeding encountered when dissecting the hilar vessels is more difficult to control if the spleen has not already been mobilized. This is especially true in the more difficult laparoscopic splenectomy.

After division of as many of the posterior peritoneal attachments as possible, the inferior pole vessels are divided (Figure 7.12). Then the central vessels and the superior pole vessels are sequentially ligated and divided (Figure 7.13). Finally the short gastric vessels are divided. The instruments for vessel ligation include Endoloops (Ethicon Endo-Surgery, Cincinnati), clips, intracorporeal and extracorporeal ties and endovascular staplers. Ties and endovascular staplers are preferable because they are less likely to be displaced by retractors than clips. The endovascular staplers are excellent but require proper dissection of the vessels and adequate-sized windows to allow safe insertion of their jaws. Adequate dissection of the vessels should be performed in case there is bleeding from the staple lines. It is dangerous to insert the endovascular stapler blindly

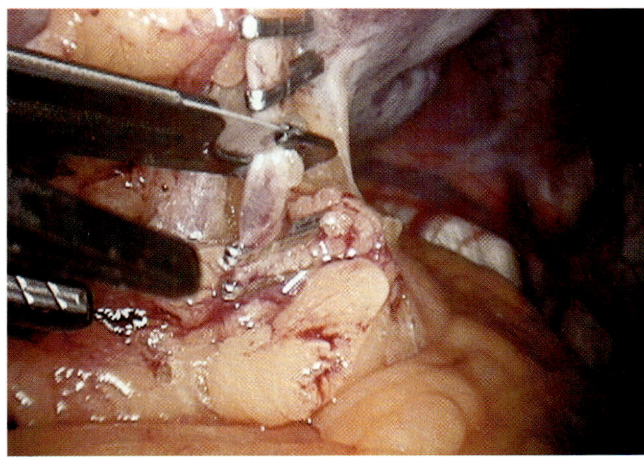

Figure 7.12: Division of splenic inferior pole vessels.

as the device may be cutting across only half of a splenic vein or artery. Proper dissection of hilar windows and careful application of the staplers is critical. However, if the spleen has been mobilized and bleeding is encountered during the dissection of the hilar vessels, the rapid application of the endovascular stapler can quickly and securely stop the bleeding in most cases.

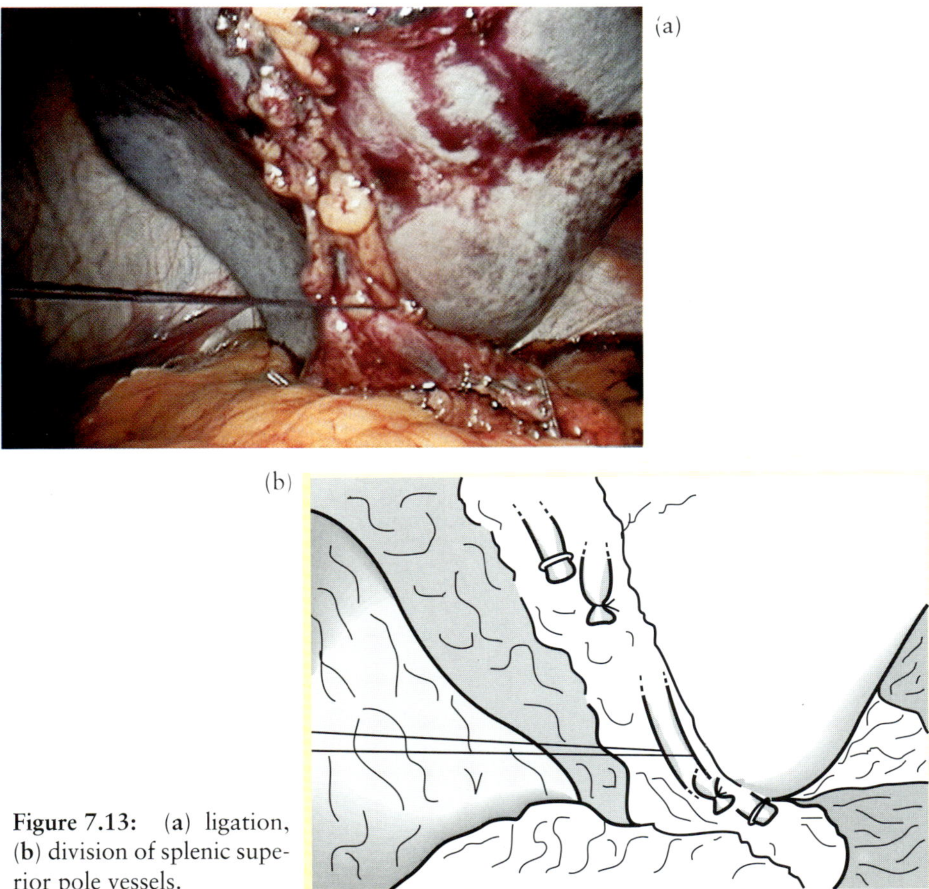

(a)

(b)

Figure 7.13: (a) ligation, (b) division of splenic superior pole vessels.

After the spleen has been detached, it is placed in a specimen bag (Cook Urologic, New Jersey) (Figure 7.14). If pathologic analysis is not crucial, the spleen can be morcellated manually with a ring forceps or mechanically at the site of the 12 mm trocar (Figure 7.15). In cases of Hodgkin's disease or other tumors that require careful pathologic analysis, the specimen can be removed intact via a lower abdominal incision. Marcaine is injected at each trocar site and the fascia is closed at each 10–12 mm trocar site (Figure 7.16).

Results

Successful laparoscopic splenectomy has been accomplished in 22 of 30 patients in whom we have attempted it. In three patients, conversion to open surgery was necessary because of bleeding. Two operations were converted because of inadequate exposure (one due to obesity and the other due to splenomegaly). Three cases were evaluated laparoscopically but were not considered candidates for laparoscopic splenectomy because of massive splenomegaly.

(a)

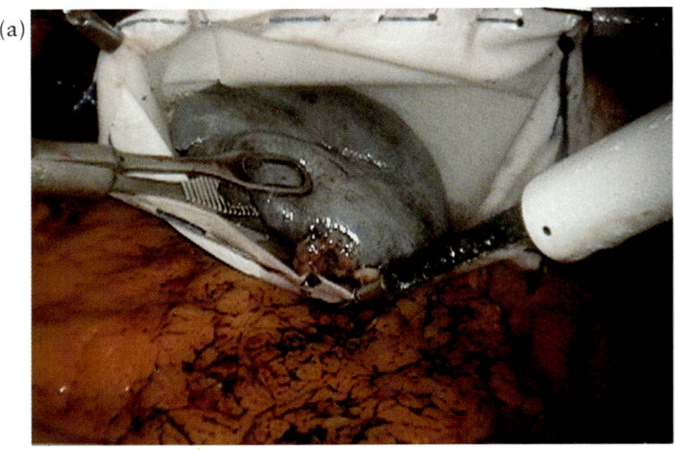

(b)

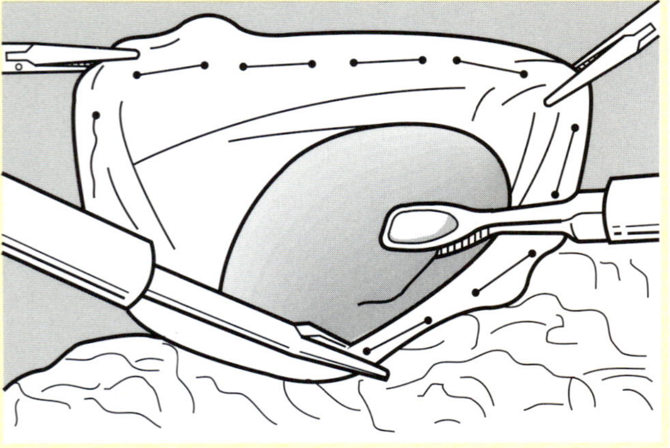

Figure 7.14: (a) detachment of the spleen, (b) placement of the spleen in a specimen bag.

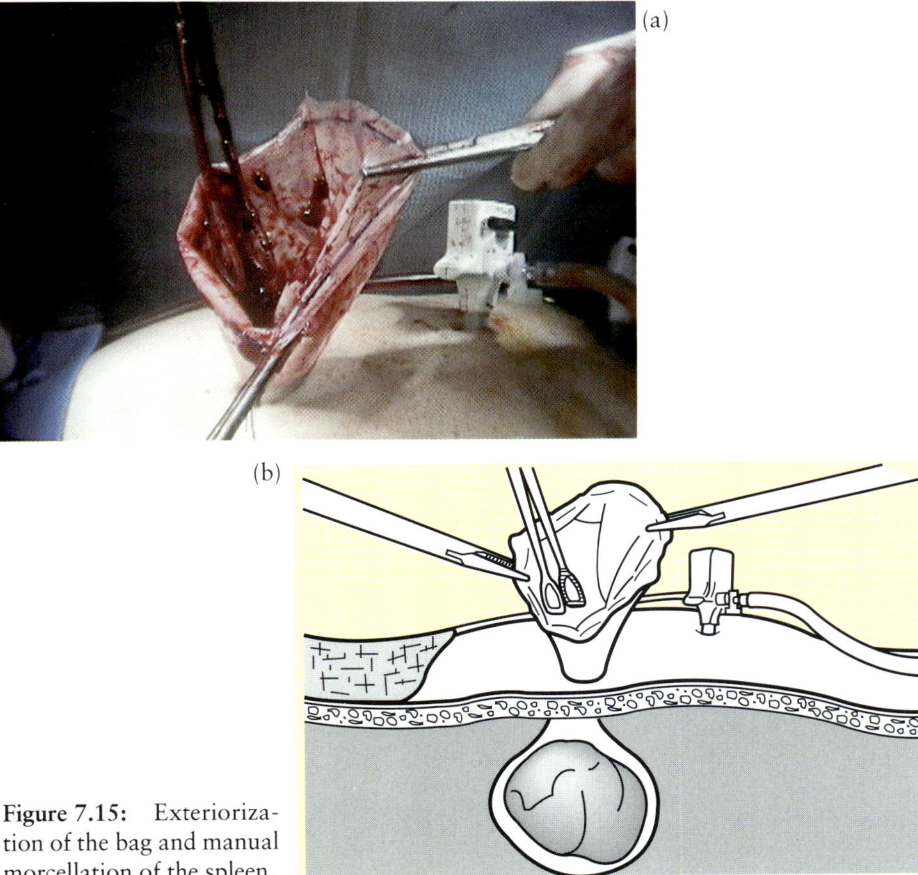

Figure 7.15: Exteriorization of the bag and manual morcellation of the spleen.

In 20 of 22 successful laparoscopic splenectomies, the spleen was removed through the 12 mm trocar site; in the two patients with Hodgkin's disease, the spleen was removed through a small lower-abdominal incision.

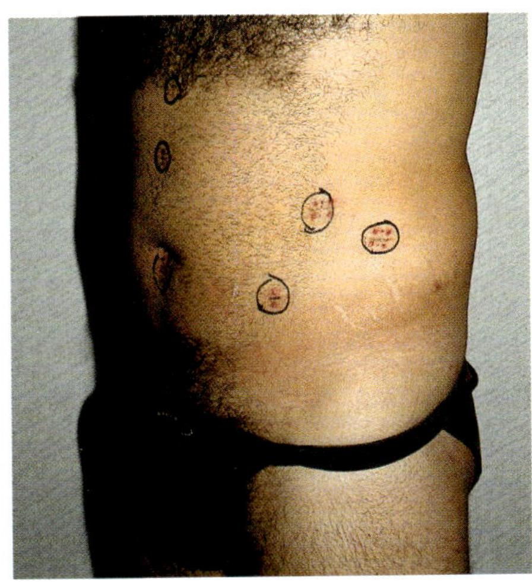

Figure 7.16: Postoperative view of trocar sites used in staging for Hodgkin's disease.

In the successful laparoscopic splenectomies, operative time averaged 144 minutes. The average blood loss was 202 cc. One patient received a transfusion of autologous blood. The average postoperative stay was 3.2 days. For the two patients with Hodgkin's disease who required an adjunctive abdominal incision for specimen retrieval, the length of post-surgical stay was four days. Oral intake was begun two days later, on average; return to driving within six days and return to work eight days after the operation. One patient had a transient seroma in his umbilical trocar site that had been significantly enlarged to remove his spleen intact.

In the larger patient group, there were three minor complications and one major complication. One patient with AIDS had a fever of unknown origin for 10 days postoperatively, and another had gross hematuria for four days following a traumatic Foley catheter insertion. One patient in the open group developed pneumonia and subsequently died of sepsis (see Table 7.2 for comparisons).

Complications

Complications following splenectomy most commonly involve the wound. Hematomas, seromas and infections occur because of coagulation abnormalities, steroid use and impaired immunity. Wound infections occur in 11% of patients who require perioperative steroids. In Musser et al.'s report[64], wound infections occurred in just 3% if splenectomy was performed for diagnostic reasons and in 6% if performed for therapeutic indications. They occasionally lead to incisional hernias, and rarely to dehiscence. The presence of a long midline or subcostal wound inevitably impairs ventilation. Pulmonary complications are common. Atelectasis is almost universal and pneumonia occurs in 7% of patients, especially in those with advanced disease.

	No Incision (n = 20)	Incision (n = 8)	Specimen incision (n = 2)
Average age	42	53	30
Average operative time (min)	144	158	172
Average blood loss (cc)	202	492	175
Average post-surgery stay (days)	2.8	9.9	4
Average return to work (days)	8.9	20.8	8
Complications			
Major	0	1	0
Minor	1	3	1

Table 7.2:   The authors' experience with laparoscopic splenectomy.

The most common intra-abdominal complication is subphrenic abscess (2%) and bleeding (2–4%). Attempts at hemostasis occasionally lead to pancreatic trauma (2%), colon injury (< 1%) and gastric perforation (< 1%). Postoperative hemorrhage (4%) is always highly morbid and is often followed by subphrenic abscess and/or pulmonary complications. Reoperation for hemostasis also increases the likelihood of serious wound complications.

Major pulmonary complications have been reported to occur in 8% of patients undergoing splenectomy[52]. Subphrenic abscess occurs in 4.2%, pancreatic injury in 2.3% and hemorrhage in 1.4%. Thromboembolic complications occur in 1.4%. In general, these complications double in incidence when splenectomy is performed for secondary hypersplenism.

Laparoscopic splenectomy is too new for us to know its true complication rate, though early results have been spectacular[83–86]. It offers the hope that the avoidance of an upper abdominal incision will lower the pulmonary complications, thromboembolic complications and wound complications associated with open splenectomy. Intra-abdominal infections may also be decreased by decreasing operative trauma, minimizing the effect on the patient's immune system and decreasing contamination of the operative site. These advantages will be offset if the incidence of operative complications and postoperative hemorrhage increase because of the complexity of the technique. Additionally, the patients who would benefit the most medically are patients with advanced Hodgkin's disease, lymphomas and leukemias. Unfortunately they invariably have significant splenomegaly. It is unclear how many of these patients will be successfully operated laparoscopically.

Conclusions

Spleen tumors, primary or metastatic, are rare compared with tumors in other parenchymal organs. Though infrequently encountered by the abdominal surgeon, they often require removal for either diagnosis or treatment. The introduction of laparoscopic surgery as an alternative approach for splenectomy has accentuated the difficulty and the challenges associated with surgery on the spleen. In our series, laparoscopic splenectomy proved to be a safe and feasible alternative to open splenectomy. The reduction in postoperative discomfort, the rapid return of bowel function and the short period of hospitalization contrasted strikingly with the same factors in patients who underwent open splenectomy. The necessity for conversion to an open operation decreased as operative experience was gained. Complications with laparoscopic splenectomy have been minimal despite the coexistence of significant comorbid illness in half of the patients.

Though only two patients with Hodgkin's disease were operated upon, they clearly benefited from the laparoscopic approach, despite the necessity for a small lower abdominal counterincision for removal of the intact spleen and additional trocars to sample the pelvic lymph nodes. Massive splenomegaly and partial splenectomy still remain outside the bounds of this technique, limiting its application in the treatment of splenic tumors. However, with improvement in instrumentation, proper patient selection, careful technique, good surgical judgement and experience in advanced procedures, it may become the standard technique for removal of spleens and their tumors in the future. Great care must be taken not to miss accessory spleens in those conditions in which residual splenic tissue would result in reactivation of the disease.

Acknowledgements

We would like to thank Drs Leon Morgenstern and Stephen Geller for their help and the use of their slides. We would also like to acknowledge the hard work of Drs Brendan Carroll and Moses Fallas; and Emma Matt for her help in preparing this manuscript.

References

1   Rosner F (1972) The spleen in the Talmud and other Jewish writings. *Bull Hist Med.* **46**: 82–5.

2   Pearson HA (1993) The spleen and disturbances of splenic function. In: Nathan and Oski. *Hematology of infancy and childhood*, vol. 2, 4th edn. W.B. Saunders, Philadelphia. pp. 1058–77.

3   Fioravanti L (1921) The treasure of human life. In: *The Spleen and some of its Diseases.* B Moynihan Wright, Bristol.

4   Virchow R (1846) Weisses blut und milztumoren. *Med Zeit.* **15**: 157.

5   Wells S (1866) On excision of enlarged spleen, with a case in which the operation was performed. *Med Times & Gaz.* **1**: 2–5.

6   Pean J (1867) Operation de splenotomie (ablation d'un kyste splenique et extirpation complète de la râte hypertropheé), guérsion. *L'union Med.* **4**: 340–4, 373–7.

7   Wells TS (1888) Remarks on splenectomy with a report of a successful case. *Proc R Med Chir Soc Lond.* **2**: 368.

8   Johnston GB (1908) Splenectomy with a review of six cases. *Johns Hopk Hosp Bull.* **19**: 178–9.

9   Wintrobe MM (1993) *Clinical Hematology*, 9th edn. Lea and Febiger, Philadelphia.

10   King H and Shumacker HB (1952) Splenic studies. I. Susceptibility to infection after splenectomy performed in infancy. *Ann Surg.* **136**: 239.

11   Morgenstern L and Shapiro S (1980) Partial splenectomy for nonparasistic splenic cysts. *Am J Surg.* **139**: 278–81.

12   Salky B *et al.* (1985) Splenic cyst—definitive treatment by laparoscopy. *Gastrointest Endosc.* **31**: 213–15.

13   Morgenstern L *et al.* (1993) Subtotal splenectomy for Gaucher's disease: a follow up study. *Am Surg.* **59**: 860–5.

14   Morgenstern L *et al.* (1985) Tumors of the spleen. *World J Surg.* **9**: 468–76.

15   Quershi MA (1964) Nonparasitic cysts of the spleen. *Arch Surg.* **89**: 570.

16   McNamara JJ *et al.* (1968) Splenic cysts in children. *Surg.* **64**: 487.

17   Fowler RH (1953) Non parasitic benign cystic tumors of the spleen. *Surg Gyn Obstet.* **96**: 209.

18   Garvin DF and King FM (1981) Cysts and non lymphomatous tumors of the spleen. *Pathol Ann.* **16**: 61.

19   Ough YD *et al.* (1981) Mesothelial cysts of the spleen with squamous metaplasia. *Am J Clin Pathol.* **76**: 666.

20   Martin JW (1958) Congenital splenic cysts. *Am J Surg.* **96**: 302.

21   Burke JS (1981) Surgical pathology of the spleen: an approach to the differential diagnosis of splenic lymphomas and leukemias. Part II. Diseases of the red pulp. *Am J Surg Pathol.* **5**: 681.

22   Chan KW and Saw D (1980) Distinctive multiple lymphangiomas of the spleen. *J Pathol.* **131**: 75.

23   Pearl GS and Nassar VH (1979) Cystic lymphangioma of the spleen. *South Med J.* **72**: 667.

24   Popper H and Thomas LB (1975) Alterations of the liver and spleen among workers exposed to vinyl chloride. *Ann N Y Acad Sci.* **246**: 172.

25   Aranha GV *et al.* (1976) Hemangiosarcoma of the spleen: report of a case and review of previously reported cases. *J Surg Oncol.* **8**: 841.

26   Alpert LI and Benisch B (1970) Hemangioendothelioma of the liver associated with microangiopathic hemolytic anemia. *Am J Med.* **48**: 624.

27   Autry JR and Weitzner S (1975) Hemangiosarcoma of the spleen with spontaneous rupture. *Cancer.* **35**: 534.

28   Chen KTK *et al.* (1979) Angiosarcoma of the spleen. A report of two cases and review of the literature. *Arch Pathol Lab Med.* **103**: 122.

29   Rokitansky (1861) Über splenome. Lehrbuch der Pathol. *Anat. Bd.* 3.

30   Rappaport H (1976) Tumors of the hematopoietic system. In: *Atlas of tumor pathology.* Armed Forces Institute of Pathology, Washington DC. pp. 91–204.

31   Long JC and Aisenberg AC (1974) Malignant lymphoma diagnosed at splenectomy and idiopathic splenomegaly. *Cancer.* **33**: 1054.

32   Farrer Brown G *et al.* (1972) The diagnosis of Hodgkin's disease in surgically excised spleens. *J Clin Pathol.* **25**: 294.

33   Vardimen JW *et al.* (1975) Malignant histiocytosis with massive splenomegaly in asymptomatic patients: a possible chronic form of the disease. *Cancer,* **36**: 419.

34   Gaba AR *et al.* (1978) Multicentric giant lymph node hyperplasia. *Am J Clin Pathol.* **69**: 86.

35   Berge T (1965) Splenoma. *Acta Pathol Microbiol Scand.* **63**: 333.

36   Cotelingam JD and Jaffe ES (1984) Inflamatory pseudotumor of the spleen. *Am J Surg Pathol.* **8**: 375.

37   Hullbert JC and Graf R (1983) Involvement of the spleen by renal angiomyolipoma: Metastasis or multicentricity? *J Urol.* **130**: 328.

38   Wick MR *et al.* (1982) Primary nonlymphoreticular malignant neoplasms of the spleens. *Am J Surg Pathol.* **6**: 299.

39   Berge T (1974) Splenic metastasis: frequencies and patterns. *Acta Pathol Microbiol Scand.* **82**: 499.

40   Govoni E *et al.* (1982) Primary malignant fibrous histiocytoma of the spleen. An ultrastructural study. *Histopathol.* **6**: 351.

41   Daftary M and Barnett RN (1971) Malignant teratoma of the spleen. *Yale J Biol Med.* **43**: 283.

42   Marymount JH and Gross S. (1963) Patterns of metastatic carcinoma in the spleen. *Am J Clin Pathol.* **40**: 58.

43   Lacher MJ (1963) Role of surgery in Hodgkin's disease. *New Eng J Med.* **61**: 113–15.

44   Goodman LS *et al.* (1947). Nitrogen mustard therapy. Use of methyl- bis-amine hydrochloride and tris-amine-hydrochloride for Hodgkin's disease, lymphosar-

coma, leukemia and certain allied and miscellaneous disorders. *JAMA*. **132**: 126–32.

45   Peters VM (1958) A study of survival in Hodgkin's disease treated radiologically. *AJR*. **79**: 114.

46   Specht L (1988) Tumour burden as the most important prognostic factor in early stage Hodgkin's disease: relations to other prognostic factors and implications for choice of treatment. *Cancer*, **61**: 1719.

47   Tubiana M *et al*. (1979) Long term results of the EORTC randomized study of irradiation and vinblastine in clinical stages I and II of Hodgkin's disease. *Eur J Cancer*. **15**: 645–57.

48   Rosenberg SA and Kaplan HS (1985) The evolution and summary results of Stanford randomized clinical trials of the management of Hodgkin's disease: 1962–1984. *Int J Radiat Oncol Biol Phys*. **11**: 5–32.

49   DeVita VT *et al*. (1970) Combination chemotherapy in the treatment of Hodgkin's advanced Hodgkin's disease. *Ann Int Med*. **73**: 881–95.

50   Glatstein E *et al*. (1969) The value of laparotomy and splenectomy in the staging of Hodgkin's disease. *Cancer*. **24**: 709–18.

51   Enright LP *et al*. (1970) The surgical diagnosis of abdominal Hodgkin's disease. *Surg Gyn Obstet*. **130**: 853–8.

52   Fabri PJ *et al*. (1974) Proceedings: a quarter century with splenectomy. Changing concepts. *Arch Surg*. **108**: 569–75.

53   Cannon WB *et al*. (1975) Staging laparotomy with splenectomy in Hodgkin's disease. *Surg Ann*. &: 103–14.

54   Ferguson DJ *et al*. (1973) Surgical experience with staging laparotomy in 125 patients with lymphoma. *Arch Int Med*. **131**: 356–61.

55   Blackledge G *et al*. (1980) Computed tomography (CT) in the staging of patients with Hodgkin's disease. A report on 136 patients. *Clin Radiol*. **31**: 143–7.

56   Carde *et al*. (1993) The EORTC H6 Trials in early stage HD. *J Clin Oncol*. **11**: 2258–72.

57   Meadows AT *et al*. (1989) Second malignant neoplasms following childhood Hodgkin's disease: treatment and splenectomy risk factors. *Med Ped Oncol*. **17**: 477–84.

58   Trueblood HW *et al*. (1970) Preservation of ovarian function in pelvic irradiation for Hodgkin's disease. *Arch Surg*. **100**: 236–7.

59   Enright LP *et al.* (1970) The surgical diagnosis of abdominal Hodgkin's disease. *Surg Gyn Obstet.* **130**: 853–8.

60   Glatstein E *et al.* (1969) The value of laparotomy and splenectomy in the staging of Hodgkin's disease. *Cancer.* **24**: 709–18.

61   Ferguson DJ *et al.* (1973) Surgical experience with staging laparotomy in 125 patients with lymphoma. *Arch Int Med.* **131**: 356–61.

62   Cannon WB *et al.* (1976) Staging laparotomy with splenectomy in Hodgkin's disease. In: Nyhus (Ed.) *Surgery Annual.* Appleton Century Crofts. New York. pp. 103–14.

63   Slavin R and Nelsen TS (1973) Complications from staging laparotomy for Hodgkin's disease. *Nat Canc Inst Monog.* **36**: 457.

64   Musser G *et al.* (1984) Splenectomy for hematologic diseases. The UCLA experience with 306 patients. *Ann Surg.* **200**: 40–5.

65   Schwartz SI (1994) Spleen. In: Schwartz, SI, Shires TG and Spencer FC (eds) *Principles of Surgery*, vol II, 6th edn. McGraw Hill, New York. pp. 1443–4.

66   Rousselot LM *et al.* (1962) Splenectomy for hypersplenism in Hodgkin's disease. A reappraisal. *Am J Surg.* **103**: 769–74.

67   Strawitz JG *et al.* (1961) Surgical aspects of hypersplenism in lymphoma and leukemia. *Surg Gyn Obst.* **112**: 89–95.

68   Neal TF *et al.* (1992) Splenectomy in advanced chronic lymphocytic leukemia: a single institution experience with 50 patients *Am J Med.* **93**: 435–40.

69   Delpero JR *et al.* (1990) Splenectomy for hypersplenism in chronic lymphocytic leukemia and malignant non-Hodgkin's lymphoma. *Br J Surg.* **77**: 443–9.

70   Damasio EE *et al.* (1990) Splenectomy after initial therapy with alpha-IFN in patients with hairy-cell leukemia (HCL): a multi-center study by the Italian Cooperative Group for HCL. Preliminary results. *Eur J Haematol.* **52** (Suppl.): 29–31.

71   Piro L *et al.* (1990) Lasting remissions in hairy-cell leukemia by a single infusion of 2-chlorodeoxyadenosine. *New Eng J Med.* **322**: 1117–21.

72   Maehara Y *et al.* (1991) Splenectomy does not correlate with length of survival in patients undergoing curative total gastrectomy for gastric carcinoma. Univariate and multivariate analyses. *Cancer.* **67**: 3006–9.

73   Brady MS *et al* (1991) Effect of splenectomy on morbidity and survival following curative gastrectomy for cancer. *Arch Surg.* **126**: 359–64.

74 Sonnendecker EW *et al.* (1989) Splenectomy during primary maximal cytoreductive surgery for epithelial ovarian cancer. *Gyn Oncol.* **35**: 301–6.

75 Phillips EH *et al.* (1993) Laparoscopic choledochoscopy and extraction of CBDS. *World J Surg.* **17**: 22–8.

76 Phillips EH *et al.* (1993) Laparoscopic preperitoneal inguinal hernia repair without peritoneal incision. *Surg Endosc.* **7**: 159–62.

77 Franklin ME *et al.* (1993) Laparoscopic colonic procedures. *World J Surg.* **17**: 51–6.

78 Phillips EH *et al.* (1992) Laparoscopic celectomy. *Ann Surg.* **216**: 703–7.

79 Carroll B *et al.* (1993) Laparoscopic cholecystectomy in critically ill cardiac patients. *Am Surg.* **59**: 783–5.

80 Cuschieri A *et al.* (1992) Technical aspects of laparoscopic splenectomy: hilar segmental devascularization and instrumentation. *J Roy Coll Surg Edin.* **37**: 414–16.

81 Lefor AT *et al.* (1993) Laparoscopic splenectomy in the management of immune thrombocytopenia purpura. *Surg.* **114**: 613–18.

82 Delaitre B *et al.* (1992) Laparoscopic splenectomy. *Br J Surg.* **79**: 1334.

83 Carroll BJ *et al.* (1992) Laparoscopic splenectomy. *Surg Endosc.* **6**: 183–5.

84 Delaitre B and Phillips EH (1993) Laparoskopische Splenektomie. In: Herausgegeben von Brune IB and Schoenleben K (eds) *Laparo-Endoskopische Chirurgie.* Hans Marseille, Munchen. pp. 273–280

85 Phillips EH (1993) Laparoscopic splenectomy. In: Hunter JG and Sackier J (eds) *Minimally Invasive Surgery.* McGraw-Hill, New York. pp 309–13.

86 Phillips EH *et al.* (1994) Laparoscopic splenectomy. *Surg Endosc.* **8**: 931–3.

8

Laparoscopic resection of the colon and rectum

BRUCE V MACFADYEN JR and CHARLES R MATHIS

Introduction

Although laparoscopic surgical techniques have been utilized for several years by gynecologists and some general surgeons, it was not until 1986 that the first video laparoscopic cholecystectomy was successfully completed[1]. This exciting technological development stimulated general and thoracic surgeons to adapt it to other abdominal and thoracic surgical procedures. While the new equipment required further surgical training because of different eye–hand coordination, the basic surgical principles were the same as in standard open procedures. The use of laparoscopic techniques in colon surgery began in 1986 when Semm performed a laparoscopic appendectomy and Gotz[2] published a large series. In his series, laparoscopic mobilization of the right colon was described in patients who had retrocecal appendicitis. Subsequently[3–5], further applications of these techniques were reported in three more small series in which the left and right colon and rectum were removed for benign and malignant disease. The use of these techniques has since expanded to include all colectomies, abdominoperineal resection, colostomy and colonic bypass.

Surgeons who perform operations for malignant disease have always stressed the importance of cancer-controlling operating techniques, and have questioned whether these principles may not be sufficiently utilized in laparoscopic colon resections because of limitations in instrumentation. Although benign disease of the colon and rectum does not lead to further spread of the disease, infection-control principles are always a concern in colorectal surgery and should not be breached. Until now there has not been a comprehensive analysis of the published data, and the purpose of this review is to address specifically the adequacy of laparoscopic surgical resection for cancer, (including lymph node resection) and local recurrence. Because these procedures have been performed for only three or four years, long-term data are not available and will require several more years to accumulate. At present, a prospective randomized trial is in progress in the USA, and these data will be presented in two or three years. This present analysis relies on retrospective information, and compares this with data from the open technique which has been accepted as the 'gold standard'. This chapter is intended to help surgeons to incorporate these procedures into clinical practice.

Surgical standards for colorectal resection

Bowel resection and the 'no-touch' technique

In open and laparoscopic colorectal surgery one must consider various issues, including the extent of the bowel resection, adequacy of lymph node removal, prevention of local recurrence, and wound implantation by malignant cells, staging of the disease, and the 'no-touch' technique. First, with regard to the extent of bowel resection, it is important to include 5 cm of proximal and distal bowel from the tumor along with the mesentery of the resected bowel including the primary arterial and venous blood supply ligated at the arterial origin. In the rectum, 5 cm of bowel proximal to the tumor and 2 cm of distal bowel and a wide mesenteric resection to the pelvic side walls and high ligation of the arterial and venous blood supply are necessary. The no-touch technique has been disputed by Wiggers *et al.*[6] who reported the results of a prospective randomized trial, comparing the no-touch isolation technique to conventional wide resection. One hundred and seventeen patients were in the no-touch group and 119 patients in the control group. It was noted that the complications were equal in both and survival was not significantly different between the two treatment groups. Although they concluded that there may be a trend toward improved survival in the no-touch group, the final analysis did not support this statistically. Therefore early ligation of the regional blood vessels during laparoscopic or open procedures is not important for cancer control.

Ligation of blood supply

Ligation of the regional arterial supply at its origin and high ligation of the venous blood supply and mesentery are also very important issues. In patients who require resection of the right colon, the distal 15–20 cm of ileum, right colon and proximal transverse colon and their mesentery should be removed. In addition, the ileocolic and right colic arteries and veins and the proximal branch of the middle colic artery and vein should be ligated and resected at their origin. For transverse colon lesions, the entire transverse colon and mesocolon along with the hepatic and splenic flexures should be removed. The middle colic artery should be ligated at its origin from the superior mesenteric artery, and there should be high ligation of the middle colic vein. Tumors in the left colon require removal of the distal transverse, left and sigmoid colon including their mesenteries. High ligation of the left colic and sigmoid arteries should be performed at their origin from the inferior mesenteric artery, along with high ligation of the corresponding veins. For proximal and middle rectal lesions, removal of the sigmoid colon, rectum and corresponding mesenteries should be performed so as to include at least 5 cm of proximal bowel and 2 cm of distal rectum. Ligation and resection of both the superior rectal artery at its origin from the inferior mesenteric artery and the middle rectal artery laterally at the pelvic sidewall should be performed. More extended bowel and lymph node resections that include periaortic lymph nodes and ligation of the inferior mesenteric artery for left-sided and rectal lesions have been considered[7]. However, Sugarbaker and Corlew[8] concluded that there is no statistically significant benefit in long-term survival.

Reporting of lymph node data

These technical considerations should be included (not merely assumed) in all reports of laparoscopic bowel surgery along with lymph node data. In most reports of laparoscopic colorectal resection, the emphasis is on the technical feasibility of bowel resection, and there is very little detail about the extent of the mesentery, the number of lymph nodes removed or the level at which the major arterial and venous blood supplies were ligated.

Over the years, the extent of lymph node resection in colorectal cancer has been recognized as an important predictor in staging and survival[9–13]. This concept has also been recognized in malignancies of the bladder, prostate gland and cervix[14]. Sugarbaker and Corlew[8] noted that extensive lymph node dissection (including the regional arterial blood supply) and periaortic lymph node resection only gave a theoretical increase of 5% in long-term survival, compared with regional lymph node resection alone. In colorectal cancer, any number of positive lymph nodes in the resected specimen indicates that adjuvant chemotherapy with and without radiation postoperatively is necessary. These additional treatments have been shown to improve long-term survival[15]. Therefore the reporting of lymph node data in laparoscopic and open colorectal surgery is very important to determine the adequacy of resection, whether further treatment is necessary, and the potential for long-term survival. Although mesenteric node recovery and pathological analysis are often variable, these data are vital and the pathologist must be thorough when looking for lymph nodes. If necessary, the pathologist must defat the mesentery to increase the nodal yield. Scott and Grace[16] emphasized this technique when they examined 41 rectal and 62 colon specimens. When traditional methods for lymph node identification were utilized, they recorded an average of 6.2 lymph nodes, whereas when a defatting procedure was used to clear the mesentery, they identified an average of 12.4 lymph nodes in each specimen. In addition, when they analyzed their data, they found that 43% of the lymph nodes obtained by traditional methods had metastases, whereas with the fat clearance technique an additional 4.8% demonstrated positive lymph nodes. This resulted in an additional 8.6% of their patients' tumor stage being changed from a Dukes' B to a Dukes' C lesion. They also compared traditional and fat clearance techniques and showed that with the defatting technique the average number of lymph nodes was 11.3 in the right colon, 6.3 in the transverse colon, 13.4 in the left colon, 13.2 in the sigmoid colon, 11.4 in the rectosigmoid, and 12.7 in the rectum (overall average 12.4 lymph nodes). With the traditional identification technique, where the average was 6.2, the right colon had the highest average number of lymph nodes (9.6 per specimen). Overall, they concluded that it was necessary to have 13 lymph nodes in the resected mesocolon or mesorectum to state that at least 90% of the nodal metastases were identified (Figure 8.1).

In a recent report by Ota *et al.*[17], the numbers of lymph nodes in standard open resected colon specimens were analyzed retrospectively in Dukes' B and C colon cancers at the M.D. Anderson Hospital. They observed that the average number of lymph nodes resected from the right colon was 18.8 ± 11.2, in the left colon resections it was 15.8 ± 16.2, and in sigmoid colon specimens 11 ± 8.6. These data were compared with specimens from laparoscopically assisted right colon resections where the average number of lymph nodes was 8.8 ± 5.4. This reduction was significant in that mesenteric lymph node resection was less adequate with the laparoscopic approach than with the traditional open operation. Vayer *et al.*[18] reported similar findings when comparing open and laparoscopically assisted colectomies. In their series the mean lymph node count was 6.6 per specimen for the laparoscopic group, which was significantly lower than the 9.6 lymph nodes per specimen in a series of open operations.

It is concluded from these data that whatever operative technique is utilized, the mesenteric resection cannot be considered adequate unless at least 13 lymph nodes have been resected. In addition, it is noted that laparoscopically assisted colon and rectal resections may not be large enough to predict local spread of disease and hence patient therapy and prognosis. Another conclusion is that when too few lymph nodes are recorded, the pathologist should use the defatting technique to maximize lymph node identification. In general, however, poor lymph node retrieval in pathological specimens is more often an indicator of inadequate surgical resection than of insufficient pathological identification.

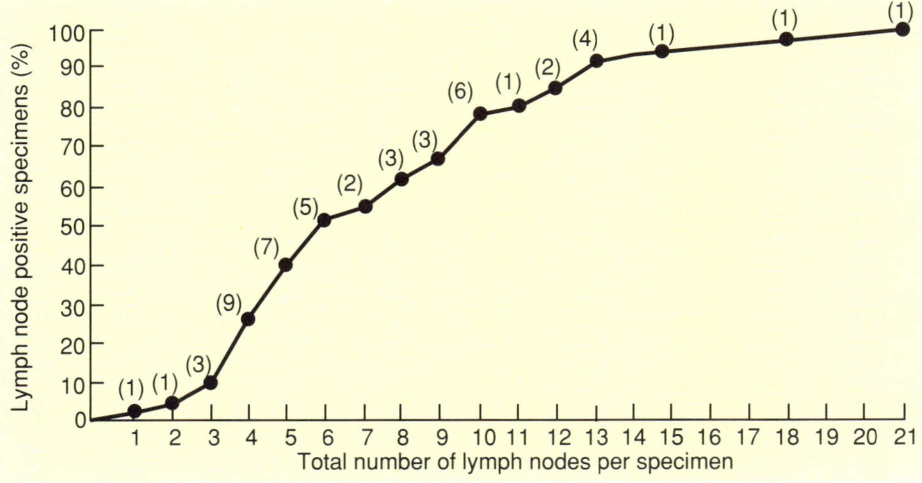

Figure 8.1:   The total number of lymph nodes recovered from each specimen, compared with the cumulative percentage of specimens which had lymph node metastases. The figures in parentheses are the actual number of specimens which yielded the given number of lymph nodes. (From Scott and Grace[16], by permission.)

Local recurrence and tumor implantation

Local recurrence after open colorectal resections has been observed. Enker *et al.*[19] found that the local recurrence rate following colon resection for Dukes' B1 and B2 malignancy was 6.9% when a 5 cm distal margin of resection was performed, as opposed to a 20% local recurrence rate when the distal margin was less than 5 cm. For patients with C2 colon cancers, they observed that an anatomical resection of the distal margin of 10 cm or more was associated with a local recurrence of 7.4% as opposed to a 36.8% local recurrence when the distal margin was less than 10 cm. Similar local recurrence rates in rectal cancer patients was noted to be 9.4% for Dukes' B1 lesions, 11.9% for B2 lesions, and 27.9% for C2 lesions. The local recurrence rate for open low anterior resection was 12.5%, compared with 24% in patients who had an abdomino-perineal resection. These data again emphasize that local recurrence is high in open colorectal surgery, and that adequate margins of bowel resection are important and must not be compromised in the laparoscopic approach. This local recurrence issue has been recorded in only one series to date[20]. Accurate recording of these data is important to assess the adequacy of laparoscopic colorectal resections.

Tumor implantation has been reported at trocar insertion sites and at the abdominal incision where the specimen was removed[21–26]. This problem may be more likely to occur when tumor extends through the serosal wall, when there is excessive manipulation of the bowel in the region of the tumor, and when a small abdominal incision is utilized to remove a large specimen. In laparoscopy, Babcock clamps and other traumatic instruments are often used to manipulate the colon and rectum, and these clamps may increase the likelihood of disruption of the bowel wall and cause tumor cells to escape intraperitoneally or at the incision site. The use of a bowel bag to remove the specimen or adhesive plastic covering of the abdominal wall incision may decrease the incidence of tumor implantation. As instrumentation improves and as surgeons increase their laparoscopic experience, this problem should become less common.

Preoperative and operative management

Assessment of the extent of tumor growth and metastasis should be carefully evaluated preoperatively. Colonoscopy is important to determine the exact location of the tumor, although sometimes the distance of the tumor from the anal verge is difficult to measure. This is particularly important when large polyps are to be excised via laparoscopic colotomy, and identification may be best obtained preoperatively with the use of India ink, methylene blue or specially prepared charcoal injected into the mucosa and submucosa via the colonoscope. In addition, the use of endoscopic ultrasound may help to determine the depth of invasion of the tumor, particularly in the rectosigmoid region. Biopsy and pathologic tumor identification can be performed through the colonoscope. Computerized axial tomography, biologic marker assays and liver function studies can also help in the staging of the disease and to determine the type of surgery to be preformed. Barium enema may be particularly helpful in laparoscopic colorectal resections because it defines the tumor location and clearly identifies the anatomy of the entire colon and rectum as the surgeon will see it intraoperatively. If one is considering doing a laparoscopic colostomy as part of the procedure, making the colostomy site on the abdominal wall preoperatively can be done with the use of indelible ink or by scratching the skin surface with a needle. A standard 24-hour preoperative bowel preparation using a purging laxative, oral antibiotics and a clear liquid diet along with a rectal suppository eight to 12 hours before surgery will mechanically cleanse the bowel and cause the bowel to contract, and therefore optimize visualization at the time of surgery.

During laparoscopy, thorough intra-abdominal evaluation must be performed just as in the open operation. The liver surface and particularly the diaphragmatic region can be evaluated when a 30–60⊃ laparoscope is used. Laparoscopic ultrasound may increase the accuracy of determining subserosal liver disease as well as pancreatic lesions and mesenteric and periaortic lymph nodes. The ovaries, cul-de-sac and other areas of peritoneal spread must be completely assessed as in the open procedure. The technical aspects of laparoscopic colorectal resections have been well described[3,27–32]. It appears from the literature and from the authors' personal experience that laparoscopic assisted colorectal resections are preferred, in order to maintain standard cancer management principles and also to expedite the surgical procedure.

At present there are two principal methods of laparoscopic colon resection. With one technique, advocated by Franklin *et al.*[27], the operation is performed completely intracorporeally, including resection of the colon and rectum and respective mesentery along with an intracorporeal anastomosis. The tumor specimen is then removed through the distal bowel using a colonoscope and snare advanced through the rectum. The second type of operation is called a laparoscopically assisted colon resection. The colon is mobilized, the mesentery and vascular supply are divided, and the bowel is resected and removed through a small abdominal incision (6–8 cm in length) that is then made over the area of the proposed anastomosis. The anastomosis is performed extracorporeally and the abdomen is closed. A low anterior resection and anastomosis is performed using the double and triple stapling techniques, and abdominoperineal resections can be done laparoscopically with a colostomy placed in the left lower quadrant.

Other intraoperative considerations include the fact that 61.6% of colorectal cancer patients have advanced but clinically curable disease at the time of surgery, while 38.4% have tumors involving all layers of the bowel wall[13]. Jeekel emphasized that 10–40% of patients undergoing surgery for colon cancer have fixation of their tumor to surrounding tissue[33] which might increase the necessity for conversion to an open procedure.

When the tumor is resected, prognostic factors include the degree of tumor differentiation with poorly differentiated tumors carrying a worse prognosis. Exophytic tumors have a better prognosis than those that are infiltrating the bowel wall or have serosal involvement. Tumor size, ulcerative growth and vascular invasion are also significant prognostic factors[33]. All of these factors indicate the importance of resecting adequate amounts of colon as well as mesentery so as to decrease the spillage of cancer cells and minimize local recurrence. These issues are not critical in benign disease but must be considered in the preoperative, operative, and postoperative assessment in patients with malignancy.

Results of laparoscopic colectomy

With each technique, accepted surgical principles and cancer control methods must be utilized when malignant lesions are resected. Table 8.1 gives an update of the laparoscopic colon data which have been reported in the management of benign and malignant lesions. Conversion from laparoscopic to open procedures has been reported to be as high as 41%[34]. In the collected series, the overall rate of conversion to an open procedure is 14.8% (Table 8.2) or 11.7% for all series of 10 or more patients. Various authors have concluded that conversion was necessary because of confusing anatomy, previous abdominal operations and adhesions, ureteral and vascular injury, enterotomy and large malignant lesions. However, the surgeon's level of experience also plays a part and the rate of conversion decreases after six to 10 cases (Figure 8.2)[36,38].

Recorded complications in these series are varied (Table 8.1). The overall morbidity ranges from 3 to 53% in series with 10 or more patients, compared with 21% in the open procedure[19]. The mortality in laparoscopic colorectal surgery from this review ranges from 0 to 3.6% compared with 2–5% in open surgery[40]. In reviewing these data, it is difficult to make a retrospective morbidity comparison because of the variability in reporting the information. This emphasizes the need for prospective randomized trials.

In this review, the average operative time was 158 minutes (range 40–310 minutes) in the series of 10 or more patients. Resumption of diet often began within 24–36 hours after surgery and hospital discharge occurred in four to six days. These findings show the potential reduction in hospital costs for patients undergoing laparoscopic colorectal resection.

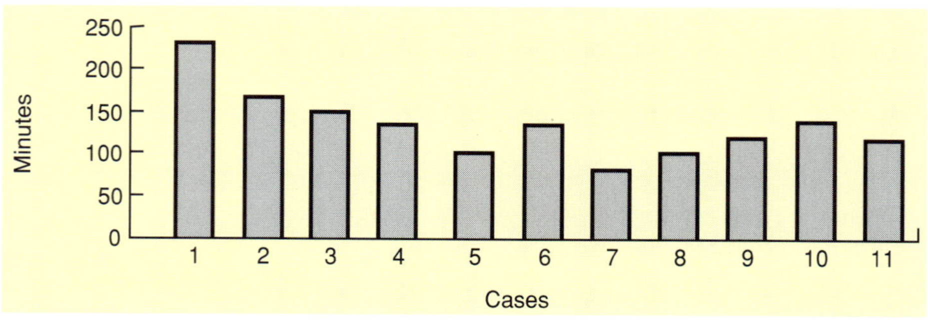

Figure 8.2:   Laparoscopic right colectomy operative time. Operative times have tended to decrease as more experience is gained. (From Peter and Bartels[36], by permission.)

In a series reporting 10 or more cancer patients with lymph node data, an average of 10.9 lymph nodes were removed (range 1–35) (Table 8.3). However, one large series reported the lymph node data of only one patient. In three series[3,30,37] which reported almost 100% of their cancer patients' lymph node results, the average number of nodes was 12.8 per specimen in this combined group (range 5–35). Table 8.1 also includes several smaller series where the emphasis was on technical feasibility, length of hospitalization, the early return to work and the low conversion rate of laparoscopic colectomy.

There is inconsistent reporting of lymph node status in cancer patients and this raises the question of the adequacy of cancer control. Therefore the emphasis on technical feasibility and the advantages to the patient (short hospitalization, early return to eating, early hospital discharge and early return to normal work activities) is really an economic issue and is not as crucial as cancer control and its effect on long-term survival.

Conclusions

Since the first description of laparoscopic colorectal surgery, it has been clear that this procedure is technically feasible. These procedures require the surgeon to be well trained in advanced laparoscopic techniques, including two-handed techniques, and intracorporeal and extracorporeal knot-tying and suturing. Laparoscopic instrumentation has greatly improved since 1991, and in the future new instruments will cause less trauma and be more efficient, further expediting the surgical procedure.

The data presented in this review indicate that the surgeon needs to perform approximately six to 10 laparoscopic colorectal operations before operative time decreases[36]. This is similar to what has been observed in other laparoscopic procedures. The importance of the surgeon being well trained in the open colorectal resection cannot be overemphasized. Laparoscopic colorectal surgical techniques should be developed and practiced in experimental laboratories and eventually utilized in patients with peer review.

For patients with malignant disease, the preferred method is the laparoscopic-assisted procedure and not the total intracorporeal operation where the specimen is removed through the distal colon. In benign disease it appears that either technique can be utilized, depending on the surgeon's skills.

The surgical management of cancer patients utilizing cancer principles cannot be overemphasized. High ligation of the blood supply along with resection of sufficient colon and rectum and necessary mesentery and lymph nodes are important cancer principles. The number of lymph nodes must be more than 12–14 per specimen; otherwise defatting pathology techniques must be utilized to determine the extent and prognosis of the disease and future treatment. Manipulation of the colon in the region of the tumor, and manipulation of the tumor itself, must not be done during the procedure, so as to decrease the possibility of local recurrence and tumor implantation at the trocar sites. The use of plastic adhesive drapes at the incision site and the use of a bag to remove the bowel may decrease the incidence of tumor implantation.

	No. of cases	Surgery	Morbidity/mortality	Conversion	Operative time (min) Average (range)	Days until resumption of diet Average (range)	Days until discharge Average (range)

Falk *et al.* (1993)[34]	66 (both cancerous and benign tumors)	Laparoscopic-assisted and laparoscopic total intra-abdominal	Major—16 (24%)
			  Enterotomies (4)
			  Splenic injuries (2)
			  Major arterial laceration (1)
			  Reoperation for bleeding (1)
			  Cerebrovascular accident (1)
			  Heart block (1)
			  Atrial fibrillation (1)
			  Anastomic dehisence (1)
			  Ileus (4)
			Minor—23 (29%)
			  Urinary tract infection (7)
			  Diarrhea (6)
			  Wound infection/hematoma (4)
			  Minor soiling (2)
			  Peristomal irritation (1)
			  Perianal irritation (1)
			  Upper respiratory infection (1)
			  Narrow anus with redundant
			    mucosa (1)
				27 (41%)	–	–	≈ 5

Franklin *et al.* (1993)[27]	91 colon resections (79 cancerous, 12 benign)	Laparoscopic total intra-abdominal and colonoscopy, left colectomy, abdominoperineal colectomy, low anterior colectomy, right colectomy, sigmoid colectomy	Morbidity—3 (3.3%) Cerebrovascular accident (1) Postoperative gastrointestinal bleeding (1) Pneumonia (1) Mortality—1 (1.1%) Death from pneumonia two days after surgery	6 (4.5%)	Right colectomy—105 Transverse colectomy—168 Left colectomy—126 Sigmoid colectomy—132 Laparoscopic-assisted—156 Abdominoperineal colectomy—105 Total 102	1 1.25 1 1 1.25 0.75 Total 1.04	2.5 3.5 2.5 3.8 3.6 2.8 Total 2.3
Jacobs *et al.* (1991)[29]	20 (11 cancerous, 9 benign)	Laparoscopic-assisted and laparoscopic total intra-abdominal, sigmoid colectomy, low anterior colectomy, right colectomy, abdominoperineal colectomy	Morbidity–3 (15%) Small bowel obstruction (1) Edematous anastomosis requiring sigmoidoscopic decompression (1) Postoperative bleeding (1)	–	170	18/20 1 day after surgery	14/20 4 days after surgery
Zucker *et al.* (1994)[3]	65 (39 cancerous, 26 benign)	Laparoscopic-assisted, right colectomy, left colectomy, abdominoperineal colectomy	Morbidity—4 (6.1%) Pneumonia (1) Urinary tract infection (1) Subfascial abscess (1) Ileus (1)	2 (3.1%)	142 (110–217)	(1–7)	4.1 (3–8)

Continued

	No. of cases	Surgery	Morbidity/mortality	Conversion	Operative time (min) Average (range)	Days until resumption of diet Average (range)	Days until discharge Average (range)
Polglase et al. (1993)[26]	8 (5 cancerous, 3 benign)	Laparoscopic-assisted, right colectomy	Morbidity—6 (75%) Wound infection (3) Congestive heart failure (1) Urinary tract infection (2)	0	133	(2–5)	10 (7–24)
Walsh et al. (1993)[23]	1 (cancerous)	Laparoscopic-assisted, right colectomy	Tumor recurrence at trocar site (1)	0	–	–	–
Scoggin et al. (1993)[35]	20 (2 cancerous, 18 benign)	Laparoscopic-assisted, right colectomy, colostomy, colotomy, sigmoid colectomy	Morbidity—4 Urinary tract infection (1) Urinary retention (1) Postoperative bleeding (1) Small bowel obstruction 2° to internal hernia(1)	0	178 (40–280)	2.3	5
Peters et al. (1993)[36]	28 (14 cancerous, 14 benign)	Laparoscopic-assisted, right colectomy, left colectomy, sigmoid colectomy, abdominoperineal colectomy	Morbidity—3 (10.8%) Ileus (1) Urinary retention (1) Urinary tract infection (1) MI (1) Mortality—1 (3.6%) Death from MI on POD 21	4 (14.3%)	168 (80–230)	–	–
Fusco et al. (1993)[25]	1 (cancerous)	Laparoscopic-assisted, right colectomy	Tumor recurrence at trocar site requiring excision (1)	0	–	–	–

Monson *et al.* (1992)[37]	40 (35 cancerous, 5 benign)	Laparoscopic-assisted, subtotal colectomy, right colectomy, left colectomy, sigmoid colectomy, abdominoperineal colectomy	Morbidity—7 (17.5%) Anastomotic leak (2) Urinary tract infection (2) Mortality—1 (2.5%) Death from MI on POD 1	(17.5%)	Right colectomy 210 (120–310) Left colectomy 240 (150–230)	–	8 (5–14)
Quattlebaum *et al.* (1993)[20]	40 (21 cancerous, 19 benign)	Laparoscopic-assisted, right colectomy, left colectomy, sigmoid colectomy	Morbidity—6 (15%) Transient late anastomotic stenosis (1) Pneumonia (1) Atelectasis (1) Traumatic bone fracture (1) Gastritis (1) Postoperative bleeding from trocar site (1)	–	(30–90)	2.5	4.1
Corbitt *et al.* (1992)[38]	18 (15 cancerous, 3 benign)	Laparoscopic-assisted, low anterior colectomy, left colectomy, right colectomy	0	3 (16.7%)	68 (45–90)	(1–3)	4 (3–6)

Continued

	No. of cases	Surgery	Morbidity/mortality	Conversion	Operative time (min) Average (range)	Days until resumption of diet Average (range)	Days until discharge Average (range)
Fowler et al. (1991)[31]	2 (cancerous)	Laparoscopic-assisted, sigmoid colectomy	Morbidity—1 Pulmonary failure Mortality—1 Death from pulmonary failure, above	0	180 (only 1 case reported)	3	6
Larach et al. (1993)[28]	5 (cancerous)	Laparoscopic-assisted, abdominoperineal colectomy	Morbidity—4 (80%) Enterotomy (1) Postoperative subcutaneous emphysema (1) Perforated duodenal ulcer (1) Pulmonary failure (1)	1 (20%)	323	4	5–14
Schlinkert (1991)[4]	2 (cancerous)	Laparoscopic-assisted, right colectomy	Mortality—1 Death from pulmonary failure	0	–	–	–
Cooperman et al. (1991)[5]	1 (benign, villous adenoma)	Laparoscopic-assisted, right colectomy	0	0	–	1	3
Kim et al. (1992)[39]	1	Laparoscopic-assisted	–	0	360	–	–

Phillips et al. (1992)[30]	51 (24 cancerous, 27 benign)	Laparoscopic total intra-abdominal, right colectomy, transverse colectomy, laparoscopic-assisted, low anterior colectomy, abdominoperineal colectomy, sigmoid colectomy, right colectomy	Morbidity—4 (7.8%) Wound infection (1) CVA (1) Bleeding from gastric ulcer (1) Pneumonia (1) Mortality—1 (2%) Death from pneumonia, above	4 (7.8%)	140	3	4.6
Total (in cases of 10 or more)	460 colon resections, 15 colotomies or 454 colorectal resections		Morbidity—71/454 (15.6%) Mortality—4/454 (1%)	53/359 (11.7%)	158 (40–310)	1.96	4.6

Table 8.1: Laparoscopic colectomy, summary data.

	Conversions	Reason for conversion (N)
Falk *et al.* (1993)[34]	27/66 (41%)	Adhesions (9) Unclear anatomy (8) Technical problems (5) Small bowel in pelvis (4) Enterotomy and bleeding (4) Abscess and obesity (3) (Some cases had several reasons to convert)
Franklin *et al.* (1993)[27]	6/91 (4.5%)	Severe adhesions (1) Extensive disease (2) Bladder invasion (2) Fistula (1)
Monson *et al.* (1992)[37]	7/40 (17.5%)	Obesity Bulky greater omentum Epiploic appendices Fixation of malignancy Difficult mobilization of tumor (Specific numbers for each cause not stated)
Phillips *et al.* (1992)[30]	4/51 (7.8%)	Inflammation from diverticulitis (2) Tumor adhesed to stomach and duodenum (2)
Corbitt (1992)[38]	3/18 (16.7%)	Unable to identify the colonic lesion laparoscopically (3)
Larach *et al.* (1993)[28]	1/5 (20%)	Enterotomy and bleeding (1)
Zucker *et al.* (1994)[3]	2/65 (3.1%)	Poor exposure (1) Ileal perforation (1)
Peters *et al.* (1993)[36]	4/28 (14.3%)	Intraoperative bleeding (1) Metastatic tumor, poorly defined anatomy (2) Enterocolonic fistula (1)
Total	54/364 (14.8%)	

Table 8.2:   Conversion of laparoscopic colectomy to open procedure.

These data indicate that laparoscopic colorectal resections can be performed with low morbidity and mortality. However, only a few papers discuss ureteral identification, although this is important in all colorectal resections.

Rates of conversion to an open operation have been reported to range from 0 to 41%. It may be important to open the patient because of confusing anatomy, adhesions, bleeding, a large malignant tumor, widespread metastases, and small bowel and ureteral injury. Patient safety is crucial and conversion should not be considered a failure on the part of the surgeon. In

	Number of patients	Number of patients with node data	Number of nodes Average (range)
Phillips et al. (1992)[30]	51 (24 cancerous, 18 benign, 9 polyps)	24	14 (8–22)
Falk et al. (1993)[34]	66 (benign or malignant)	Sigmoid colectomy—5 Right colectomy—8	8 (3–13) 13 (3–25)
Franklin et al. (1993)[27]	91 (79 cancerous, 12 benign)	1	14
Jacobs et al. (1991)[29]	20 (11 cancerous, 9 benign)	6	17.9 (8–35)
Quattlebaum et al. (1993)[20]	40 (20 cancerous, 20 benign)	1	7
Fowler et al. (1991)[31]	2 (cancerous)	2	10 (7–13)
Larach et al. (1993)[28]	4 (cancerous)	4	4.75 (1–8)
Peters et al. (1993)[36]	28 (14 cancerous, 14 benign)	–	Right colectomy—9.0 Sigmoid colectomy 7.3
Scoggin et al. (1993)[35]	20 (2 cancerous, 18 benign)	2	8.5 (7–10)
Fusco et al. (1993)[25]	1 (cancerous)	1	11
Walsh et al. (1993)[23]	1 (cancerous)	1	7
Zucker et al. (1994)[3]	65 (39 cancerous, 26 benign)	31	Right colectomy 28.4 (18–35) Sigmoid colectomy 8 (6–10) Laparoscopic-assisted 7.3 (5–11)
Monson et al. (1992)[37]	40 (35 cancerous, 5 benign)	35	10 (5–21)
Total		121	10.9 (1–35)

Table 8.3:   Lymph nodes in cancer patients.

complicated case management, early conversion may expedite the procedure and decrease potential morbidity, mortality and operative time.

These data also show that operative time is much the same as in open operations, and early oral feeding and hospital discharge can occur along with an early return to normal living activities. These factors are important economic considerations, but they are not as important as maintaining operative cancer principles and potentially improving long-term patient survival. Up till now most of the data have concentrated on technical feasibility and the economic advantages of laparoscopic colorectal resections rather than the basic principles of cancer surgery. In the future, what will be needed is long-term controlled randomized studies so that the clinical surgeon can understand the application of these procedures in his or her surgical practice.

References

1   Dubois F *et al.* (1989) Cholecystectomy par coelioscopie. *Presse Med.* **18:** 980–2.

2   Gotz F (1988) Die endoskopische Appendektomie Nach Semm bei der akuten und appendicitis. *Endoskopie heute.* **2:** 5.

3   Zucker KA *et al.* (1994) Laparoscopic-assisted colon resection. *Surg Endosc.* **8:** 12–18.

4   Schlinkert RT (1991) Laparoscopic-assisted right hemicolectomy. *Dis Colon Rectum.* **34:** 1030–1.

5   Cooperman AM *et al.* (1991) Laparoscopic colon resection: a case report. *J Laparoendosc Surg.* **1:** 221–4.

6   Wiggers T *et al.* (1988) No-touch technique in colon cancer: a controlled prospective trial. *Br J Surg.* **75:** 409–15.

7   Grinnell RS (1966) Lymphatic block with atypical and retrograde lymphatic metastasis and spread in carcinoma of the colon and rectum. *Ann Surg.* **163:** 272–80.

8   Sugarbaker PH and Corlew S (1982) Influence of surgical techniques on survival in patients with colorectal cancer: a review. *Dis Colon and Rectum.* **25:** 545–57.

9   Wolmark N *et al.* (1986) The prognostic value of the modifications of the Dukes' C class of colorectal cancer. *Ann Surg.* **203:** 115–322.

10   Dukes CE and Bussey HJR (1958) The spread of rectal cancer and its effect on prognosis. *Br J Cancer.* **12:** 309–20.

11   Copeland EM *et al.* (1968) Prognostic factors in carcinoma of the colon and rectum. *Am J Surg.* **116:** 875–81.

12   Dunning EJ *et al.* (1951) Carcinoma of the rectum: a study of the factors influencing survival following combined abdominoperineal resection of the rectum. *Ann Surg.* **133:** 166–73.

13 Spratt JS and Spjut HJ (1967) Prevalence and prognosis of individual clinical and pathologic variables associated with colorectal carcinoma. *Cancer.* **20**: 1976–85.

14 Cady B (1984) Lymph node metastasis: indicators but not governors of survival. *Arch Surg.* **119**: 1067–72.

15 Steele G (1992) Adjuvant therapy for patients with colon and rectal cancer: clinical indications for multimodality therapy in high-risk groups and specific surgical questions for future multimodality trials. *Surgery.* **112**: 847–9.

16 Scott KWM and Grace RH (1989) Detection of lymph node metastasis in colorectal carcinoma before and after fat clearance. *Br J Surg.* **76**: 1165–7.

17 Ota DM *et al.* (1994) Controversies regarding laparoscopic colectomy for malignant disease. *1994 Seminars Laparosc Surg.* (In press.)

18 Vayer AJ *et al.* (1993) Cost effectiveness of laparoscopically assisted colectomy. Personal communication.

19 Enker WE *et al.* (1979) Enhanced survival of patients with colon and rectal cancer is based upon wide anatomic resection. *Ann Surg.* **190**: 350–7.

20 Quattlebaum JK *et al.* (1993) Laparoscopically assisted colectomy. *Surg Lap Endosc.* **3**: 81–7.

21 Clair DG *et al.* (1993) Rapid development of umbilical metastasis after laparoscopic cholecystectomy for unsuspected gallbladder carcinoma. *Surgery.* **113**: 355–8.

22 Fong Y *et al.* (1993) Gallbladder cancer discovered during laparoscopic surgery: Potential for iatrogenic tumor dissemination. *Arch Surg.* **128**: 1028–32.

23 Walsh DCA *et al.* (1993) Subcutaneous mets after laparoscopic resection of malignancy. *Aust NZJ Surg.* **63**: 563–5.

24 O'Rourke N *et al.* (1993) Tumor in oculation during laparoscopy. *Lancet.* **342**: 368–9.

25 Fusco MA and Paluzzi MW (1993) Abdominal wall recurrence after laparoscopic assisted colectomy for adenocarcinoma of the colon. *Dis Colon Rectum.* **36**: 858–61.

26 Polglase AL *et al.* (1993) Laparoscopic assisted right hemicolectomy with Valtrac Bar (Biofragmentable Anastomotic Ring) Ileotransverse anastomosis. *Aust NZJ Surg.* **63**: 481–4.

27 Franklin ME *et al.* (1993) Laparoscopic colonic procedures. *World J Surg.* **17**: 51–6.

28   Larach SW *et al.* (1993) Laparoscopic assisted abdominoperineal resection. *Surg Lap Endosc.* **3**: 115–18.

29   Jacobs M *et al.* (1991) Minimally invasive colon resection (laparoscopic colectomy). *Surg Lap Endosc.* **1**: 144–50.

30   Phillips EH *et al.* (1992) Laparoscopic colectomy. *Ann Surg.* **216**: 703–7.

31   Fowler DL and White SA (1991). Laparoscopy-assisted sigmoid resection. *Surg Lap Endosc.* **1**: 183–8.

32   Wexner SD and Johansen OB (1992) Laparoscopic bowel resection: advantages and limitations. *Ann Med.* **24**: 105–10.

33   Jeekel J (1987) Can radical surgery improve survival in colorectal cancer? *World J Surg.* **11**: 412–17.

34   Falk PM *et al.* (1993) Laparoscopic colectomy: a critical appraisal. *Dis Colon Rectum.* **36**: 28–34.

35   Scoggin SD *et al.* (1993) Laparoscopic-assisted bowel surgery. *Dis Colon Rectum.* **36**: 747–50.

36   Peters WR and Bartels TL (1993) Minimally invasive colectomy: are the potential benefits realized? *Dis Colon Rectum.* **36**: 751–6.

37   Monson JRT *et al.* (1992) Prospective evaluation of laparoscopic-assisted colectomy in an unselected group of patients. *Lancet.* **340**: 831–3.

38   Corbitt JD (1992) Preliminary experience with laparoscopically-guided colectomy. *Surg Lap Endosc.* **2**: 79–81.

39   Kim LH *et al.* (1992) Laparoscopic-assisted abdominoperineal resection with pull-through (sphincter saving). *Surg Lap Endosc.* **2**: 237–40.

40   Goligher J (1981) Results of operations for large bowel cancer. In: De Cosse JJ (ed.) *Large Bowel Cancer.* New York, Churchill Livingstone. pp. 154–165.

9

Laparoscopic resection of adrenal masses

DAVID M ALBALA and RICHARD A PRINZ

Introduction

The diagnosis and management of disorders of the adrenal gland are among the most challenging and satisfying aspects of general surgical and urologic practice. Only within the past three decades have accurate diagnosis, precise radiologic localization, satisfactory preoperative medical management, appropriate anesthesia, and refined surgical techniques come together to render the surgical management of adrenal abnormalities a safe endeavor with a predictable outcome.

Virtually every conceivable approach to the adrenal gland has been recommended. Each method has advantages and disadvantages. For normal-sized or hyperplastic glands and tumors up to 5 cm the posterior approach has been recommended, but this route is inadequate for removing larger lesions. Moreover, when bilateral adrenalectomy is required, two separate incisions are needed. The advantage of this approach is that the peritoneal cavity is not entered, so ileus is unusual and the postoperative course is much less complicated. The widest exposure to the adrenal gland is offered by the lateral or transthoracic route. This approach is used for large tumors, but only one adrenal gland can be removed at a time. Associated intraperitoneal disease is not easily evaluated with this technique. The anterior or transabdominal approach allows the surgeon to evaluate both adrenal glands before removal. This has been the preferred method for removal of pheochromocytomas, as bilateral, extra-adrenal or malignant disease can easily be evaluated and appropriately treated.

Unfortunately, substantial morbidity is associated with conventional open procedures, and present-day approaches for adrenalectomy are far from perfect. Conventional operative methods also cause substantial postoperative pain, disfigurement and prolonged convalescence.

Despite its wide use by gynecologists for many years, laparoscopy has only recently been taken up by other specialists for diagnostic and therapeutic purposes. Now laparoscopy is being used increasingly, not only for primary diagnosis, but also to evaluate the extent of disease or clinical stage. Within the past five years, laparoscopic techniques have been developed and applied to: cholecystectomy, herniorraphy, pelvic lymphadenectomy, and nephrectomy[1–4]. This chapter will review our current indications, technique, and results in performing laparoscopic adrenalectomy.

Indications

There is little disagreement that conventional surgical techniques should be used in patients with large (greater than 6 cm) functioning adrenal neoplasms; however, smaller functioning and non-functioning masses may be treated with laparoscopic methods which allow their removal in a minimally invasive way. Functioning abnormalities, such as Cushing's syndrome due to an adrenal adenoma or bilateral cortical hyperplasia, aldosteronoma, and pheochromocytoma may be successfully managed with laparoscopy. Recently Gagner and associates managed a patient with Cushing's disease after failed transphenoidal hypophysectomy with bilateral laparoscopic adrenalectomy[5]. This approach gave a successful outcome with less patient discomfort and morbidity than conventional surgical techniques.

Opinions concerning non-functioning tumors are not unanimous, since less is known about their natural history. The number of these tumors removed surgically has increased in the past three or four years, mainly because of serendipitous detection by computerized tomography (CT). This has similarly contributed to the incidental detection of cysts, adenomas and hematomas[6]. Laparoscopy can be used to manage these lesions with minimal patient morbidity.

Our current indications for laparoscopic adrenalectomy include nonfunctioning adenomas that are increasing in size or suspected of causing local symptoms, pheochromocytomas, Cushing's adenoma, aldosteronomas, angiomyolipomas and medullary cysts of the adrenal gland. The laparoscopic approach for malignant adrenal neoplasm is controversial. It may be used in selected patients with lesions less than 6 cm where the risk of tumor spillage is minimal. It has been performed successfully in one patient with bilateral malignant pheochromocytomas associated with a multiple endocrine neoplasia (MEN-IIB) syndrome[7]. This patient had a previous total thyroidectomy for medullary thyroid cancer with associated features such as megacolon and large adenomatous lips.

Contraindications

Laparoscopy should be avoided in patients at high risk for bowel injury, or in those who have medical illnesses that may be exacerbated by the pneumoperitoneum. These include patients with peritonitis, extensive adhesions from multiple prior surgical procedures, mechanical or functional bowel obstruction, large intra-abdominal masses, uncorrected coagulopathy, severe cardio-pulmonary disease and hypovolemic shock.

Laparoscopic resection may be contraindicated for lesions located on the right side, when the mass is located behind the vena cava or when the right lobe of the liver extends down over the lesion. It is difficult in these cases to get enough retraction to allow adequate exposure of the adrenal mass. Laparoscopic resection may be contraindicated when an extra-adrenal extension is present. This can usually be identified by CT and radionuclide scans. Signs of extensive malignancy, such as invasion into surrounding structures or ingrowth into the vena cava, also preclude this approach. Invasion into surrounding structures and obvious malignant states are contraindications to laparoscopic methods of removal, but these minimal access techniques may be valuable in diagnosis and defining the extent of disease.

Patient preparation

Preoperative management of hormone-producing adrenal tumors is the same as with conventional, open adrenalectomy. The blood pressure of patients with pheochromocytoma is adequately controlled by preoperative administration of alpha-1 blockers. All patients require a full mechanical and antibiotic bowel preparation to help decompress the intestines and increase exposure during dissection, and to allow for conservative repair of any inadvertent bowel injury. Patients are given a broad-spectrum antibiotic before the procedure. Autologous blood should be available for transfusion if necessary.

Surgical technique

A general endotracheal anesthetic is used. Controlled ventilation is necessary to ensure adequate oxygenation and to avoid hypercarbia. Nitrous oxide can cause bowel distention and should be avoided. A nasogastric tube is placed to keep the stomach and bowels decompressed, and a Foley catheter is positioned to drain the bladder before initiating the pneumoperitoneum. Patients are placed in a lateral decubitus position for insufflation (Figure 9.1). The CO_2 insufflation is initiated in the subcostal area with a Verres needle and the abdomen is insufflated to 15 mmHg.

If adequate Verres needle position is unobtainable in the decubitus position, a Verres needle or Hasson trocar can be placed in the umbilicus and the abdomen insufflated. This will ensure an adequate pneumoperitoneum, and accessory trocars can then be placed without complication. However, this technique is more time-consuming.

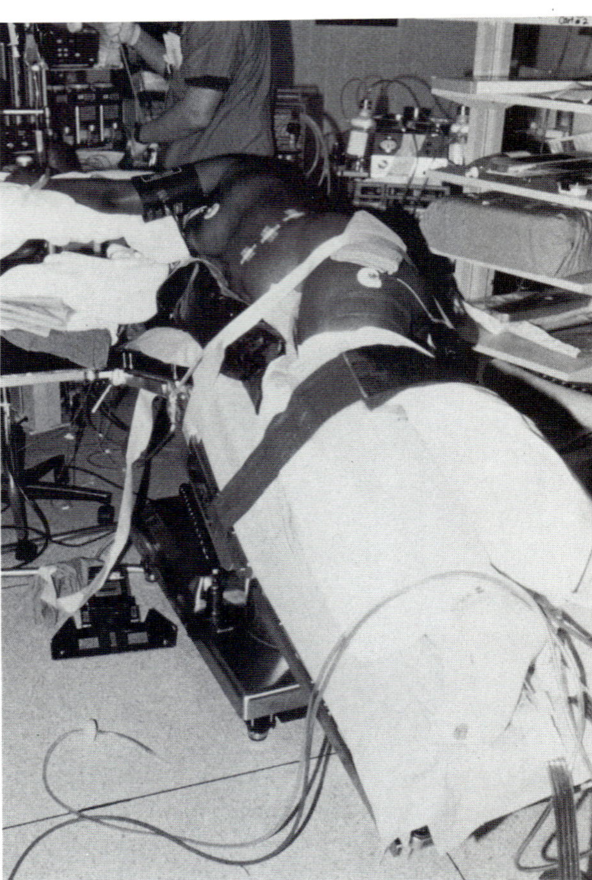

Figure 9.1: Patients are placed in the lateral decubitus position for both Verres needle and trocar placement.

Left laparoscopic adrenalectomy

After adequate insufflation of the abdomen, a 10/11 mm trocar is inserted in the left subcostal area at the level of the anterior axillary line. A 30° angled laparoscope is inserted through this trocar. Three more 10/11 mm trocars are inserted under direct vision in the flank (under the 12th rib) and dorsally (Figure 9.2). Mobilization of the splenic flexure of the colon is accomplished using endoscopic scissors to open the retroperitoneal space between the spleen and the lateral portion of the abdominal wall. The patient may also be moved to a Fowler position to permit downward migration of the bowel loops and gravity retraction of other extra peritoneal structures. The upper pole of the left kidney is exposed by freeing the posterolateral attachments of the spleen in the direction of the diaphragm. The spleen is retracted medially and superiorly with a fan or balloon retractor. The left adrenal gland should come into view at this point. The superior aspect of the adrenal gland is dissected first before the dissection is carried medially. The inferior phrenic arterial branches are ligated with titanium clips after mobilization of the superior pole.

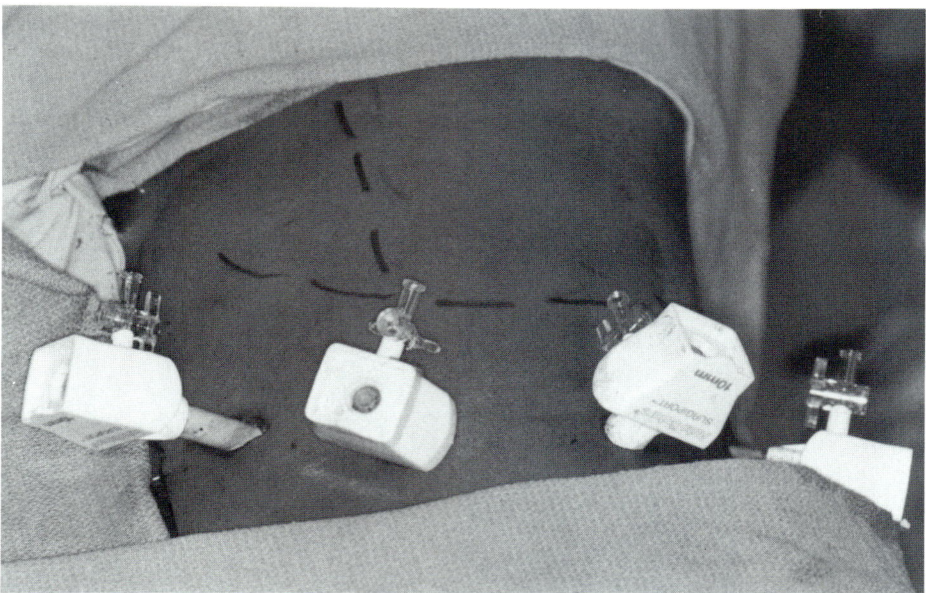

Figure 9.2:   The initial 10/11 mm trocar is placed in the left subcostal area at the level of the anterior axillary line. Three more 10/11 mm trocars are inserted under direct vision in the flank and dorsally.

The left adrenal vein is then dissected free and ligated with at least two clips (Figure 9.3). The inferior portion of the adrenal gland is dissected last and the gland separated from the surrounding tissue. Hemostasis is verified by removing all blood and clots with an irrigation/aspiration device. The gland is extracted after placement into an entrapment sac and the bag removed through the most inferior trocar site with minimal spreading of the oblique muscles and using a Kelly clamp. The trocar incision may have to be extended to remove larger tumors. All of these large trocar sites require a fascial closure. We prefer to use 2-0 vicryl suture for this. The skin edges are reapproximated according to each surgeon's preference; we use a subcuticular closure with a 4-0 vicryl suture. A long-acting local anesthetic is injected at each trocar site.

Right laparoscopic adrenalectomy

After adequate insufflation using a Verres needle or the Hasson technique as described above, the entire abdomen should be tympanitic after the pneumo-peritoneum surrounds the liver. Care must be taken during lateral insufflation to avoid placement of the Verres needle into the liver parenchyma or hepatic flexure of the colon. A 10/11 mm trocar is inserted in the anterior axillary line and used to pass the laparoscope. Two additional 10/11 mm trocars are inserted in the right flank under direct vision. The final trocar is inserted

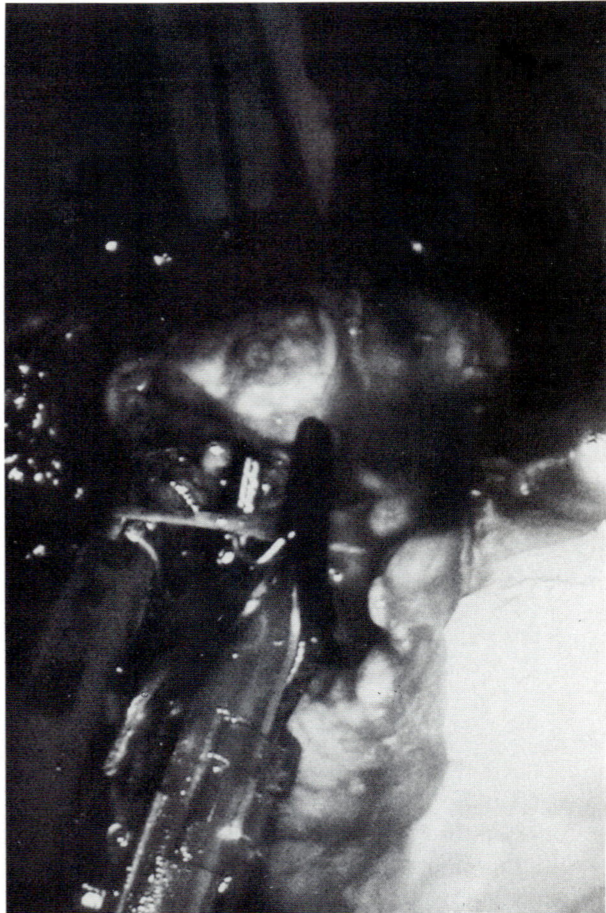

Figure 9.3:   The adrenal vein is isolated and two clips are applied. Note the adrenal mass and the fan retractor in the background.

dorsally after the retroperitoneal space has been entered and the kidney identified. The right triangular ligament of the liver is dissected free with electrocautery scissors, exposing the inferior vena cava. A fan or balloon retractor is then placed underneath the liver to retract it superiorly and medially. The patient may also be placed in a Fowler's position to allow downward migration of the bowel and fluid. The perinephric fat is dissected superiorly and close to the inferior vena cava to expose the adrenal gland. Dissection begins at the superior pole and anterior aspect of the right adrenal gland. Small vessels are secured with titanium clips and divided. A laparoscopic Kittner dissector is used to retract the medial aspect of the gland. Meticulous dissection in this area will prevent tears from lateral branches of the vena cava. The adrenal vein is isolated and at least two secure clips are placed before transecting it. The inferior pole of the adrenal gland is dissected last. When all attachments have been divided, an entrapment sac is used to remove the adrenal gland through the anterior trocar site. All large trocar sites require fascial closure and the skin edges are reapproximated. A long-acting anesthetic is injected at each trocar site before a light dressing is applied.

Postoperative care

The nasogastric tube and Foley catheter may be removed in the recovery room. Sequential stockings are left in place until the patient is ambulatory. Oral fluids are begun on the day of surgery, if tolerated. Patients resume regular activities as tolerated. Some adrenal disorders necessitate hormonal support, and this is begun in the immediate postoperative period.

Results

Eight patients (three females and five males) have undergone laparoscopic adrenalectomy at the Loyola University Medical Center. This procedure was successful in all but one case: this patient was converted to an open procedure due to bleeding from the inferior vena cava. There were no deaths in this series. None of the patients experienced respiratory or circulatory difficulties during surgery. The results for left and right laparoscopic adrenalectomy are shown in Tables 9.1 and 9.2. For the entire series, the mean operative time was 3 3/4 hours and the estimated blood loss was 385 cc. Patients remained in the hospital for an average of 2.3 days. In the immediate postoperative period, patients required an average of two doses of Meperidine hydrochloride totalling 135 mg. Complete convalescence was noted within 10 days.

The only complication in this series was bleeding from the vena cava, resulting in the need to convert to open surgery; no other vascular or bowel injuries were noted. Five right and three left adrenalectomies were performed. The mean lesion size was 4.25 cm (range 3.3–7 cm).

	Mean	Range
Time in operating room	3 h 46 min	3 h 20 min–4 h
Estimated blood loss	250 cc	150–400 cc
Hospital stay	2.67 days	1–4 days
Post-operative Demerol		
No. of doses	2	2
Dosage	125 mg	100–150 mg
Convalescence period	11 days	7–16 days

Table 9.1:   Results of laparoscopic left adrenalectomy in three patients.

	Mean	Range
Time in operating room	4 h 10 min	3 h–5 h 40 min
Estimated blood loss	540 cc	250–750 cc
Hospital stay	2 days	1–4 days
Post-operative Demerol		
No. of doses	2.25	2–3
Dosage	144 mg	100–225 mg
Convalescence period	8.5 days	6–14 days

Table 9.2:   Results of laparoscopic right adrenalectomy in five patients.

Discussion

Adrenalectomy may be indicated for a variety of disorders of the adrenal gland. Traditionally, selection of the surgical approach has been determined by size of the lesion, malignant potential, and functional state of the lesion to be removed, as well as by body habitus. The options available to the surgeon have included the retroperitoneal approach through either a flank or posterior incision, a transabdominal approach, or a thoraco-abdominal incision. Gagner and associates were the first to report the laparoscopic adrenalectomy technique in patients with Cushing's disease and pheochromocytoma[8]. This demonstrated conclusively that laparoscopic techniques could be used successfully to remove adrenal tissue. The advantages of this minimal access approach are decreased postoperative pain, minimized physical disfigurement, and the shortened convalescence period.

Access to the adrenal gland can be obtained easily with the laparoscope. The procedure is essentially the same as with open transperitoneal surgery except that laparoscopic adrenalectomy requires a smaller surgical field. Precise dissection of the adrenal gland can be carried out with the magnified view provided on the video monitor. Small vessels that are usually mass-ligated during open surgery are clearly recognizable and can be cut following precise clip application.

The flank approach for insufflation and dissection probably results in the need for less dissection than the anterior laparoscopic approach[8]. This is especially true on the left side where the tail of the pancreas has to be retracted medially and loops of bowel may come into the surgical field. With the patient in the decubitus position, the intraperitoneal organs are shifted medially. The creation of a pneumoperitoneum in this position can be performed safely, although care should be taken during insufflation to avoid Verres needle placement in the colon on both sides and in the liver parenchyma on the right side.

In our series, the operative times for right adrenalectomy tended to be approximately 25 minutes longer than those for left adrenalectomy. This increased operative time is due to the need for particularly careful dissection around the vena cava. We found this dissection difficult, and great care is needed to avoid injury to the accessory vessels of the vena cava or the cava itself. This is contrary to the experience of Go and associates who found left-sided lesions more difficult than right-sided lesions because of the necessity to retract both the left colon and pancreas[9].

Retroperitoneoscopy with CO_2 has been used by a number of urologists. In 1978 Wickham used this technique to remove a ureteral stone[10]. Kerbl and associates reported on the retroperitoneal approach for laparoscopic nephrectomy[11]. They noted that a significant amount of time was spent changing the patient's position from supine to a lateral decubitus after the pneumoperitoneum had been established. In the porcine model, they were able to remove the kidney with an entirely retroperitoneal approach. The operative time was increased, as delays were caused by using fluoroscopy to guide the Verres needle into the retroperitoneum and for initial trocar placement, and because the entrapment sac had to be opened within the confined space of the retroperitoneum.

A retroperitoneal laparoscopic nephrectomy was performed on a 48-year-old man with a chronically obstructed non-functioning kidney. The retroperitoneal approach provided excellent exposure for dissection of the renal hilum but human anatomic factors limited port placement and organ entrapment. They also noted an increased risk for the development of a pneumothorax[11]. Recent reports have suggested that use of a balloon catheter may alleviate some of the problems encountered with the retroperitoneal approach[12]. This approach has not been used yet on the adrenal gland although it may allow for easier dissection.

This small series demonstrates the wide range of endocrine disorders of the adrenal gland that may be treated laparoscopically. The disadvantages of this approach include: (1) longer operative time, (2) risk of vascular and internal organ injuries, (3) complications due to pneumoperitoneum from using CO_2 and (4) higher operative cost than with open surgery because of the disposal instruments. The advantages of this approach over standard adrenalectomy are the same as with other laparoscopic procedures, ie less postoperative discomfort, less disfigurement and a shorter hospital stay.

In conclusion, laparoscopic adrenalectomy is a safe alternative method for removal of adrenal masses that is useful for all types of adrenal lesions except malignant disease. Further studies are required with malignant disease because of the risk of disseminating malignant cells into the abdominal cavity. Although the operative times are somewhat lengthy, these problems should be overcome as techniques are improved and new laparoscopic instruments are introduced.

References

1 Reddick EJ and Olsen DO (1989) Laparoscopic laser cholecystectomy. *Surg Endosc.* **3**: 118–20.

2   Popp LW (1990) Endoscopic patch repair of inguinal hernia in a female patient. *Surg Endosc.* **5**: 10–13.

3   Winfield HN *et al.* (1992) Laparoscopic pelvic lymph node dissection for genitourinary malignancies: indications, techniques, and results. *J Endourol.* **6**: 103–11.

4   Albala DM *et al.* (1992) Laparoscopic nephrectomy. *Sem Urol.* **3**: 146–51.

5   Gagner M *et al.* (1992) Laparoscopic adrenalectomy in Cushing's syndrome and pheochromocytoma. *New Engl J Med.* **327**: 1003.

6   Hattery RR *et al.* (1981) Computed tomography of the adrenal gland. *Semin Roentgenol.* **16**: 290–300.

7   Gagner M *et al.* (1993) Early experience with the laparoscopic approach for adrenalectomy. *Surgery.* **114**: 1120–5

8   Gagner M *et al.* (1993) Laparoscopic adrenalectomy. *Surg Endosc.* **7**: 122–4

9   Go H *et al.* (1993) Laparoscopic adrenalectomy for primary aldosteronism: a new operative method. *J Lap Surg.* **3**: 455–9

10   Wickham JEA (1979) The surgical treatment of renal lithasis. In: *Urinary Calculous Disease.* Churchill Livingstone, New York. pp. 145–98

11   Kerbl K *et al.* (1993) Retroperitoneal laparoscopic nephrectomy: laboratory and clinical experience. *J Endosc.* **7**: 23–5

12   Gaur DD (1990) Laparoscopic operative retroperitoneoscopy: use of a new device. *J Urol.* **148**: 1137–9

10

Laparoscopic placement of enteral feeding tubes

DAVID M OTA and STEVEN STANDIFORD

Introduction

Laparoscopic surgery is being adapted for abdominal procedures that previously required an open laparotomy approach. Cholecystectomy, appendectomy, colectomy and Nissen fundoplication can be performed with minimal access techniques. These laparoscopic methods represent an advance in abdominal surgery because incisions ≤ 1 cm mean that postoperative recovery is faster, with shorter hospitalization, less incisional pain and an earlier return to normal activity.

A number of minimal access techniques have recently been developed to establish routes for enteral feeding. Percutaneous endoscopic gastrostomy (PEG) is now employed routinely, but is associated with reflux[1]. Percutaneous endoscopic jejunostomy has recently been described[2,3], involving the passage of either a long pediatric endoscope or balloon catheter to identify the proximal jejunam and then puncturing the bowel wall percutaneously with catheter insertion over a guide wire[2]. Similar techniques have been developed by invasive radiologists who can place feeding tubes under fluoroscopic guidance. However, negotiating the duodenum can be difficult and patients with a strictured pylorus or duodenum related to malignant disease are not good candidates for this procedure. Consequently a technique of laparoscopic jejunostomy tube placement was developed to access the proximal gastrointestinal tract for enteral feeding when endoscopic procedures were not feasible.

Patient selection

Patients with upper gastrointestinal malignant diseases are potential candidates for laparoscopic enteral feeding tubes. Such patients may have considerable nutritional deficits and require nutritional support in order to complete a planned course of therapy such as radiotherapy or chemotherapy. If a PEG or fluoroscopic tube placement is not feasible and nutritional supplements are necessary, a laparoscopic gastrostomy or jejunostomy tube placement should be considered. There are several clinical scenarios in which a laparoscopic feeding tube may be needed. Locally advanced esophageal carcinoma can produce a long stricture that may preclude passage of a pediatric endoscope or a fluoroscopically placed percutaneous gastrostomy tube. If radiotherapy or combined chemoradiotherapy are being considered, a laparoscopically placed feeding tube may offer a solution for gaining enteral access. Advanced gastric carcinomas are being treated with preoperative chemotherapy that can produce significant gastrointestinal side-effects[4]. Here again a potential rate limiting factor in completing the therapy is the nutritional status of the patient. Carcinoma involving the head of the pancreas is being treated with preoperative chemoradiotherapy[5,6]. Considerable data are available to show that this can prolong survival and can better control loco-regional disease after resection[6]. Because the malignant disease and upper abdominal radiotherapy can result in significant anorexia, placement of jejunal feeding tubes is necessary. While duodenal or jejunal tubes can be placed by endoscopic or fluoroscopic means, they often migrate back into the stomach or cannot be placed beyond the duodenal loop because of tumor distortion. In these instances, laparoscopic methods to insert enteral feeding tubes distal to the tumor site provided an attractive alternative. If abdominal radiotherapy is going to be administered, the jejunostomy tube feeding site should always be placed outside the field of radiotherapy. For patients with pancreatic carcinoma another important advantage of laparoscopy is intra-abdominal staging. A significant number of these patients will have peritoneal pathology discovered at the time of laparoscopy[7].

Another clinical scenario in which laparoscopic enteral feeding tubes may be beneficial is trauma. Injured patients who require diagnostic laparoscopy[8] or general anesthesia for head, facial or orthopedic blunt injuries may require enteral feedings postoperatively. The advantage of a jejunal feeding tube is that the incidence of aspiration is lower than with a gastrostomy tube, especially in the presence of head trauma. While patients should not be given a general anesthetic solely for enteral feeding, the laparoscopic procedure may be appropriate if other surgical procedures require anesthesia.

Methods

The first method involves the laparoscopically assisted jejunostomy tube placement[9]. The port sites, location of TV monitor, and position of the surgeon and assistant are shown in Figure 10.1. The laparoscope is placed in the camera port (10 mm) located at the infraumbilical site. Other 5 mm port sites are placed as shown. If the patient has malignant disease, then the abdominal cavity is explored systematically. The patient is placed in the reverse Trendelenburg position. The left and right lobes of the liver are examined for metastatic nodules. The left and right diaphragm are inspected for plaques that may represent carcinomatosis and should be biopsied. The anterior surface of the

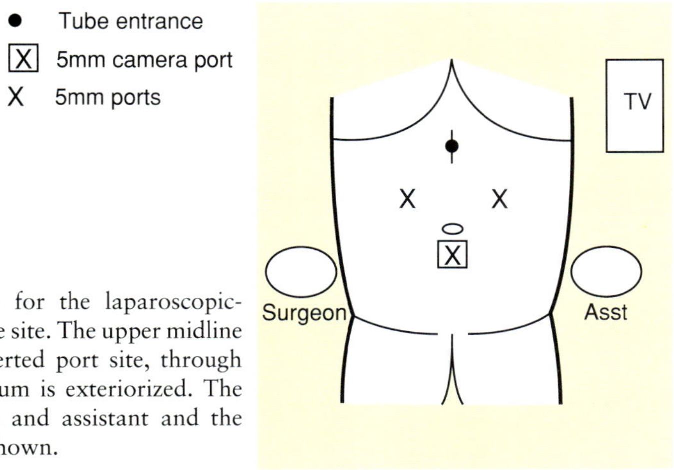

Figure 10.1: Port sites for the laparoscopic-assisted jejunostomy tube site. The upper midline 3 cm incision is a converted port site, through which the loop of jejunum is exteriorized. The position of the surgeon and assistant and the video monitor are also shown.

stomach and the underside of the left lobe of the liver are visualized, then the left and right paracolic gutters and greater omentum are examined. The patient is then placed in the Trendelenburg position. The greater omentum is gently lifted out of the pelvis and placed cephalad to the transverse colon. The rectal cul-de-sac, bladder and uterus are examined. Peritoneal washings with 0.9% NaCl irrigant are taken for cytology.

The next step is to identify the ligament of Treitz. The mid-transverse colon is gently grasped and lifted with a grasper in the right port. Occasionally the mesentery may have to be grasped. A grasper in the left port is used to trace the bowel in the left upper quadrant to the ligament of Treitz. On some occasions the ligament may not be obvious, but when the small bowel is traced to a segment that cannot be pulled caudad, the proximal jejunum has been found. This is because the proximal jejunum is fixed at the ligament of Treitz while the remaining small bowel is very mobile. If there is any doubt about the location of the proximal jejunum, the laparoscopic approach should be abandoned. Reasons for not being able to find the ligament include excessive adhesions from previous surgery and diffuse carcinomatosis.

Once the proximal jejunum has been found, a segment which is 20–30 cm from the ligament of Treitz is grasped through the upper midline port. A 2–3 cm midline incision is made at this port and the jejunal loop is exteriorized (Figure 10.2). If a gastrostomy tube is needed, the greater curvature of the stomach can be grasped and exteriorized through this small incision. The Witzel jejunostomy tube placement is now completed extracorporeally. The 3–0 silk pursestring suture is placed and the tube is advanced 15–20 cm through the enterotomy. A silastic 12–14 Fr tube is preferred. The pursestring suture is tied and a series of interrupted Lembert sutures is placed over the tube to create a serosal wrap (Figure 10.3). The jejunal loop is pushed back into the abdominal cavity and the jejunostomy site is sutured to the peritoneum on one side. The fascia is closed around the tube using interrupted sutures. The skin is closed and the feeding tube is anchored to the skin with a monofilament suture.

Postoperative recovery is rapid. Pain control can be achieved with oral medications or elixir preparations via the feeding tube. If pain control is adequate, the patient can be discharged from the recovery room or kept

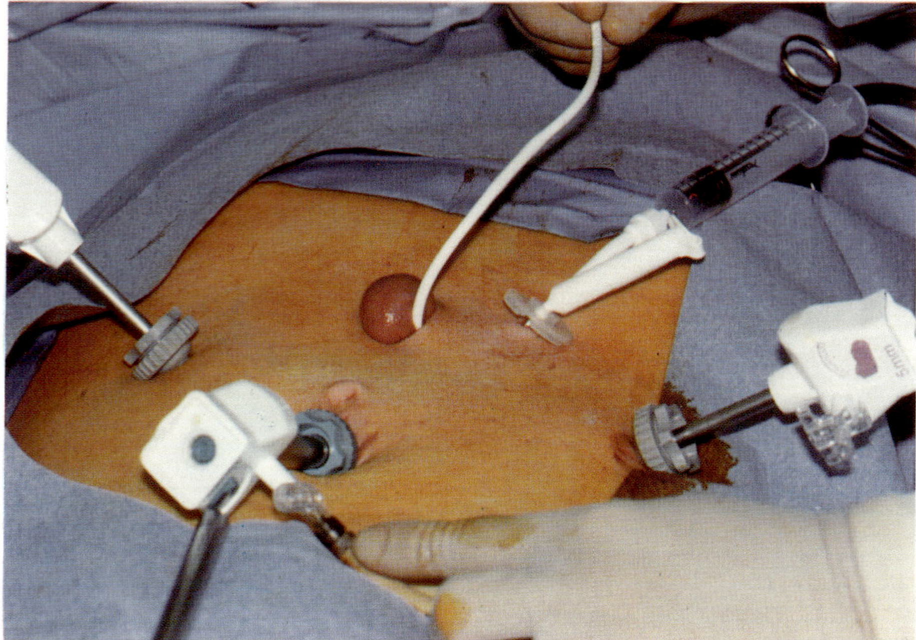

Figure 10.2: Exteriorized jejunal loop, from the left leg looking up toward the right shoulder. Once the loop of jejunum is exteriorized, the tube is inserted through the pursestring suture.

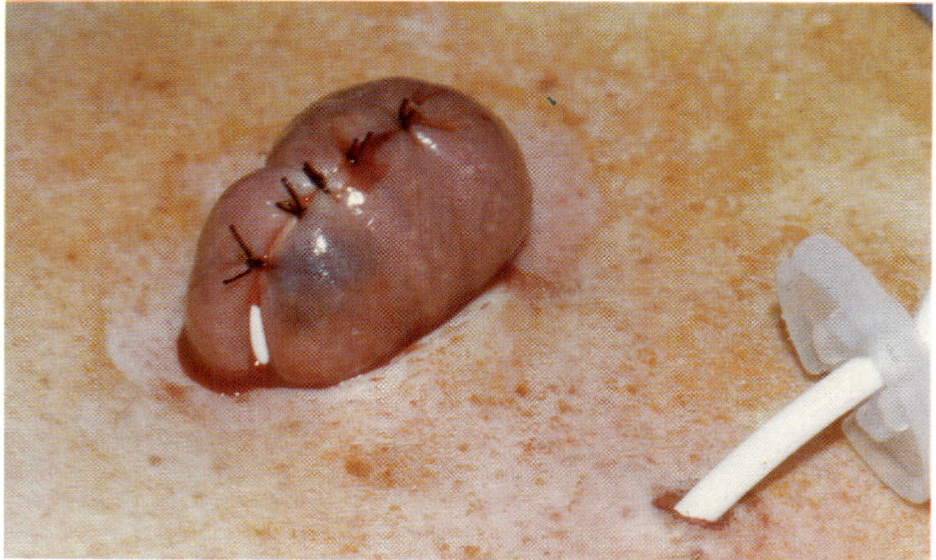

Figure 10.3: The serosal wrap is completed for the Witzel jejunostomy tube. The loop jejunum is then gently pushed back into the abdominal cavity and sutured up to the anterior abdominal wall through the small incision.

overnight. Tube feeding can begin the next day as an outpatient using an ambulatory enteral feeding pump at 45 mL/h and a full-strength tube feeding product. The feedings can be advanced to 65–85 mL/h the following day. Continuous feedings up to 125 mL/h are usually tolerated.

The next phase of development deals with intracorporeal suturing of the Witzel jejunostomy tube: can the entire Witzel procedure be done within the abdominal cavity? The completely intracorporeal laparoscopic jejunostomy technique was developed in a canine model, and followed exactly the same principles as the open technique. Eight dogs underwent laparoscopic jejunostomy; all procedures were successful, with no episodes of small bowel leak, and there was secure anchorage of the enterostomy site to the abdominal wall in all cases at postmortem examination. This preclinical information became the basis for conducting a prospective clinical trial.

The method of an intracorporeal Witzel jejunostomy tube placement is based on our animal studies. The patient is placed in a supine position. Under general anesthesia, one camera and two operating ports are placed as shown in Figure 10.4. The infraumbilical port is for the laparoscope. The surgeon and assistant stand on the right side and the video monitor is placed on the patient's left side. The jejunostomy tube site is in the left upper quadrant. This positioning aligns the surgeon, suturing site and video monitor in a straight line and offers maximum comfort to the surgeon's arms. The abdomen is explored as described previously for the laparoscopic-exteriorized method. Once the proximal jejunum is identified (Figure 10.5), a 3 mm stab incision is made in the left upper quadrant with a #11 scalpel blade. A 3–0 Nylon on a Keith needle is passed into the abdominal cavity through the stab incision. Figure 10.6 shows the Keith needle entering the abdominal cavity as seen through the laparoscope. The proximal jejunal loop is brought up to the needle, which is passed through the antimesenteric side of the bowel (Figure 10.7). It is important to spear the bowel to the side of the antimesenteric edge so that the bowel faces the surgeon and laparoscope. A 14 G needle is passed through the stab incision into the peritoneal cavity. The Keith needle is grasped with a laparoscopic needle holder and inserted into the 14 G needle which is used to guide the Keith needle out of the abdominal cavity through the stab incision (Figure 10.8). Docking the

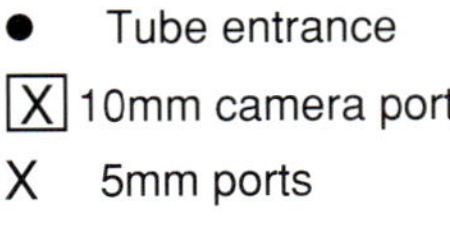

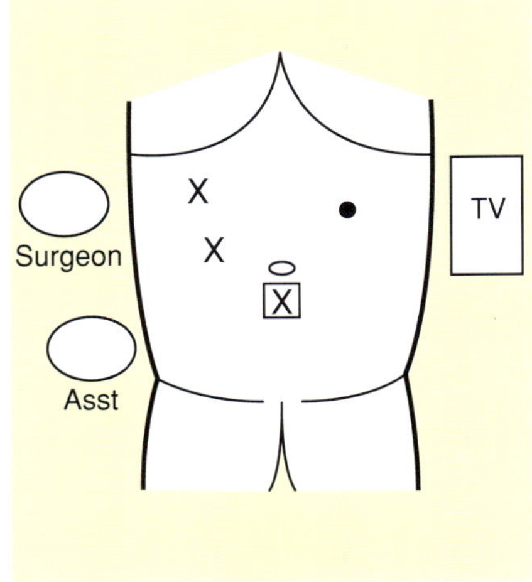

Figure 10.4:   Port sites for the intracorporeal feeding jejunostomy technique. Both the surgeon and the assistant stand on the right side and the video monitor is placed on the patient's left side. The jejunostomy tube site is in the left upper quadrant.

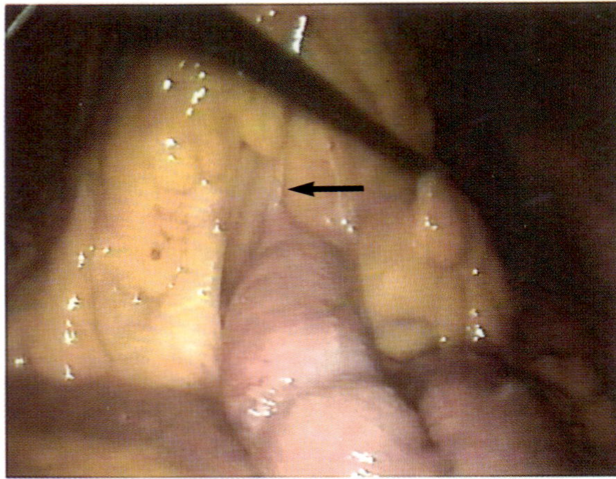

Figure 10.5: Infraumbilical port site, looking towards the upper abdomen. The greater omentum has been lifted over the transverse colon. The transverse colon is lifted upwards and the proximal jejunum is attached to the base of the transmesocolon. Arrow shows the ligament of Treitz.

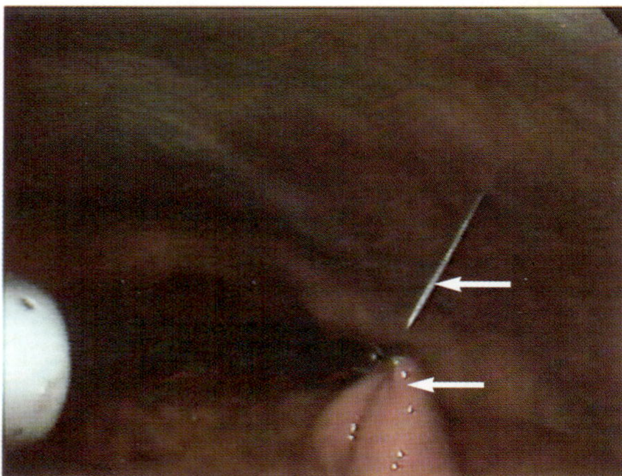

Figure 10.6: The Keith needle (*arrow*) has been passed through a 3 mm stab incision into the abdomen in the left upper quadrant, and the proximal jejunal loop (*arrow*) had been brought up to the needle.

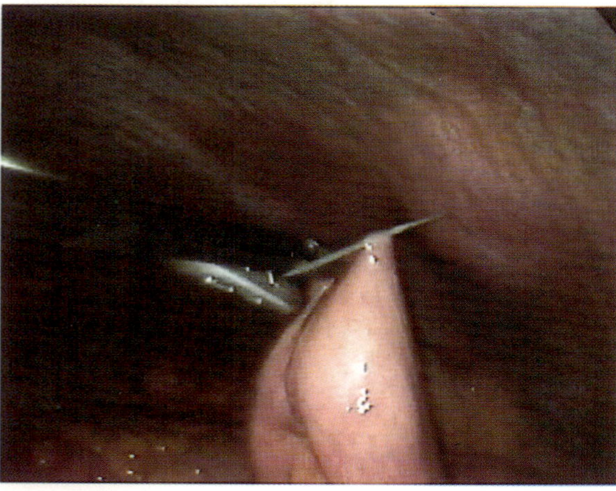

Figure 10.7: The needle has been passed through the side of the antimesenteric edge of the bowel. The needle and suture are pulled through with the laparoscopic needle-holder.

Keith needle with another needle is necessary to bring the suture out through the stab incision. Once the needle is out, the 3–0 Nylon is tied below the stab incision and cut. The 3–0 Nylon should be tied securely such that the proximal bowel is now anchored to the anterior abdominal wall. This suture has two functions. First, fixation of the bowel to the anterior wall greatly facilitates

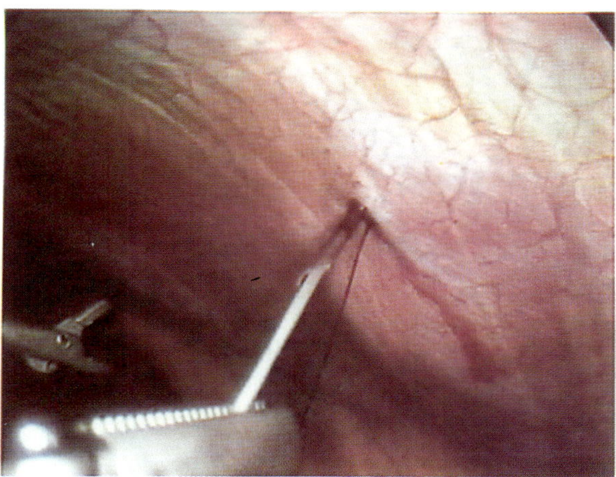

Figure 10.8: The 14 G needle has been passed into the abdominal cavity through the stab incision. The Keith needle is then inserted into the 14 G needle and passed out of the abdominal cavity. The needle-in-needle maneuver guarantees that the needle and suture exit through the 3 mm stab incision.

suturing because the suturing site is always kept before the surgeon and laparoscope. Secondly, this suture fixes the jejunostomy site to the abdominal wall. The passage of the Keith needle out of the abdominal cavity through the stab incision with the 14 G needle allows the surgeon to place the knot below the skin. Placement of this knot below the skin avoids any routine postoperative visit for suture removal.

When the jejunal loop has been fixed to the anterior abdominal wall, the distal limb should be facing the laparoscope and surgeon (Figure 10.9). A 3–0 Vicryl suture on a ski-needle (20 cm long) is passed into the abdominal cavity through the right lower port with a laparoscopic needle holder. The Szabo-Berci needle-holder and goose-neck grasper (Karl Storz) are helpful in performing the intracorporeal suturing. A four-point pursestring suture is placed on the distal limb. The tail end of the suture should only be 1–1.5 cm long (Figures 10.10, 10.11).

A Russell gastrostomy kit is used to obtain a 10 mL syringe, 15 cm needle, guide wire, three dilators and a peel-away sheath. A Silastic or polyurethane 12-Fr nasogastric tube is cut to 30 cm in length. A 5 mm stab incision is made near the anchoring stitch. The needle on the air-filled syringe is inserted through the incision into the peritoneal cavity. Under laparoscopic observation the

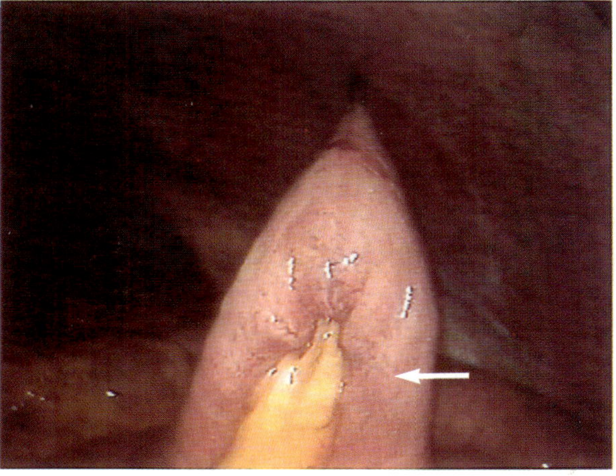

Figure 10.9: The loop of jejunum is fixed to the anterior abdominal wall after the 3–0 Nylon suture has been tied below the skin level. The distal limb is to the right (*arrow*). The Keith needle has been placed slightly off the antimesenteric line, and the antimesenteric border is therefore now facing the laparoscope and surgeon.

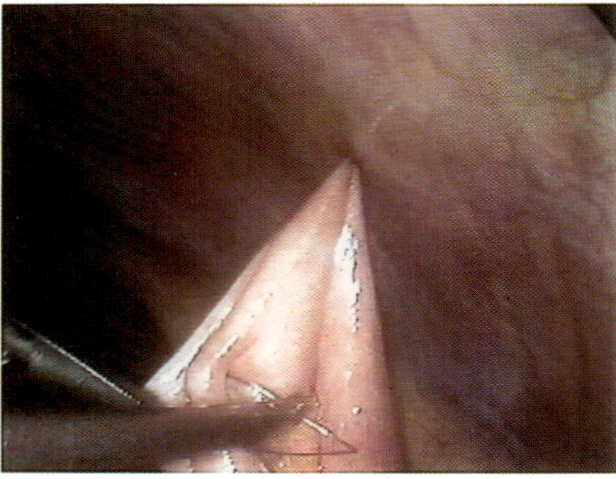

Figure 10.10: Initial stitch of a 3–0 Vicryl suture (15 cm length) on a ski-needle, for the pursestring suture on the distal jejunal limb.

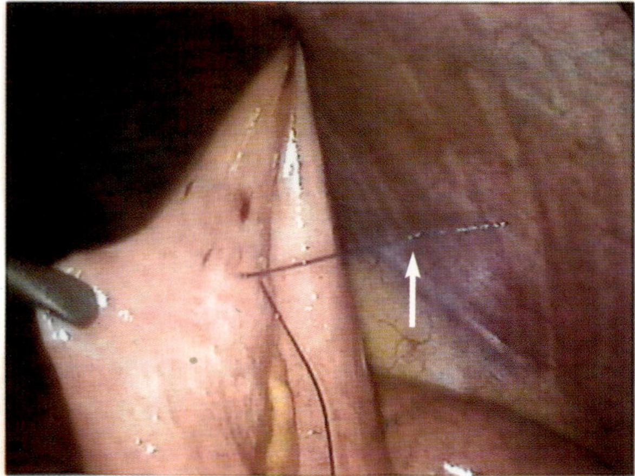

Figure 10.11: The pursestring suture has been completed with a short end, 1.5 cm long (*arrow*).

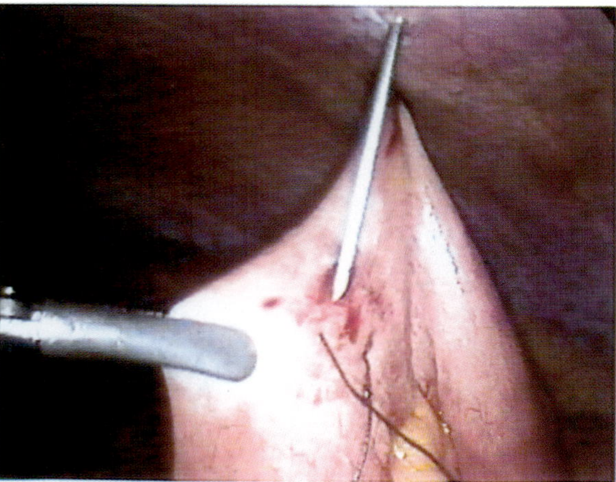

Figure 10.12: The needle has been passed into the abdominal cavity and through the center of a pursestring suture. Air is insufflated through this needle to determine if the needle is in the lumen of the bowel.

needle is inserted into the center of the pursestring suture as shown in Figure 10.12. Air is inserted to check that the needle tip is in the bowel lumen. The syringe is removed and the guide-wire is inserted through the needle into the bowel lumen. The wire can be passed into the distal lumen for 15–20 cm with gentle manipulation of the bowel using a grasper (Figure 10.13). The needle is removed and enlarging dilators are passed over the wire into the bowel. The peel-away sheath is inserted over the wire and the dilator is removed (Figure 10.14). The feeding tube is inserted through the peel-away sheath over the guide-wire. The wire is removed and the sheath is peeled away (Figure 10.15).

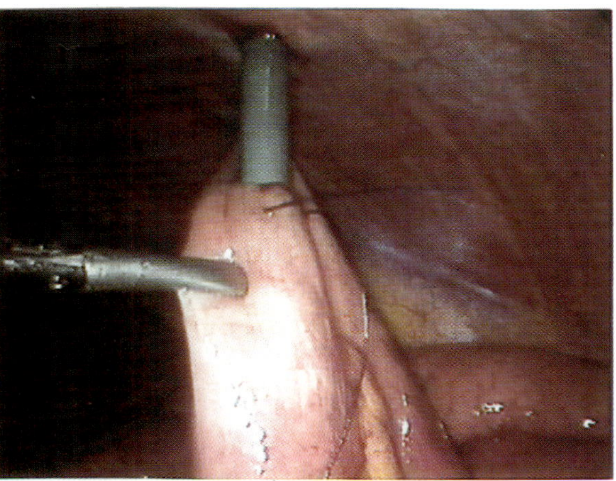

Figure 10.13: The guide-wire has been passed through the needle and down into the distal limb of jejunum. The needle is removed and all that remains is the guide-wire.

Figure 10.14: Peel-away sheath in place. After the three dilators have been placed and removed, a peel-away sheath and dilator are inserted over the guide-wire through the pursestring suture into the bowel lumen.

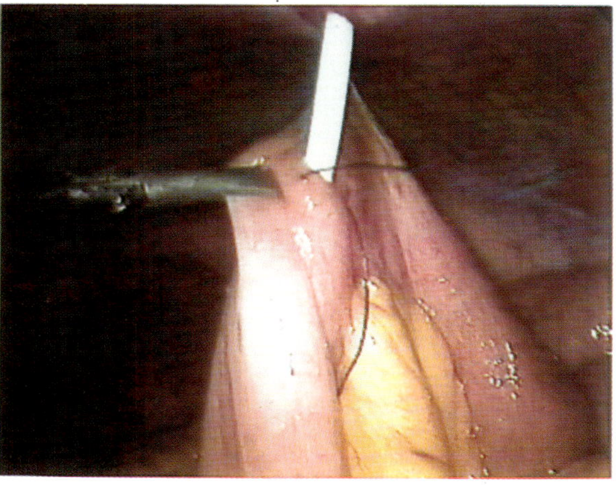

Figure 10.15: The feeding tube is passed approximately 20 cm over the guide-wire through the peel-away sheath into the jejunum. The guide-wire is pulled out. The peel-away sheath is then removed and, as shown here, the 12 Fr feeding tube is put into place.

Next a laparoscopic needle-holder and goose-neck grasper are used to tie the pursestring with three throws as depicted in Figure 10.16. Only the short end is cut. The needle and suture for the pursestring is now used to create a serosal wrap around the feeding tube (Figure 10.17). Two or three running Lembert sutures are placed. These sutures should be carefully placed to avoid an excessive serosal tunnel that can compromise the jejunal lumen. A 12-Fr feeding tube is suitable for this and allows the use of inexpensive intact protein formulas. A Lapra-Ty (Ethicon, Inc.) suture clip is passed through the right lower port and a grasper through the right upper port pulls on the suture as the Lapra-Ty is applied. The Lapra-Ty acts like a split-shot tie and has a lock–snap mechanism. Once applied to the suture, the Lapra-Ty holds the suture and therefore also the serosal wrap (Figure 10.18). The needle is then passed through the peritoneum in two places and secured each time with a Lapra-Ty (Figure 10.19). The jejunostomy site is now anchored in three places (Figure 10.20). The feeding tube is sutured to the skin with 3–0 Nylon. The CO_2 is removed and the port sites are closed with a subcuticular closure. The patient can be discharged from the recovery room. Because there is no incision management, all postoperative care can be done by telephone. This procedure can also be adapted to put a Witzel gastrostomy tube in place. The anterior

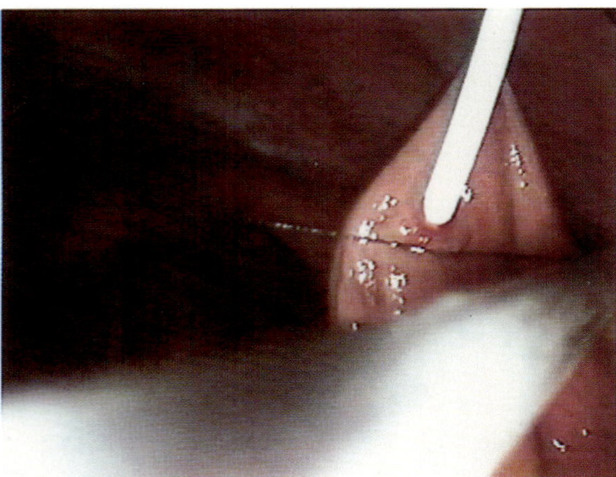

Figure 10.16: The pursestring suture is then tied using intracorporeal instrument tying technique. The suture is tied three times and only the short end is cut. The remaining suture is used to create the serosal tunnel.

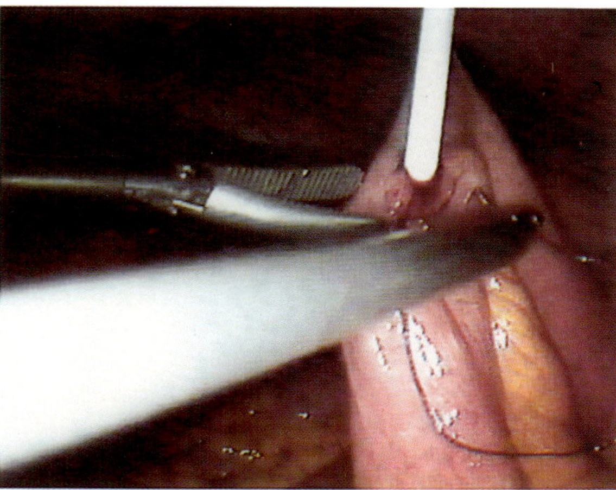

Figure 10.17: The remaining Vicryl suture on the ski needle is then used to create a serosal wrap around the feeding tube. A continuous Lembert stitch is used to create this serosal tunnel.

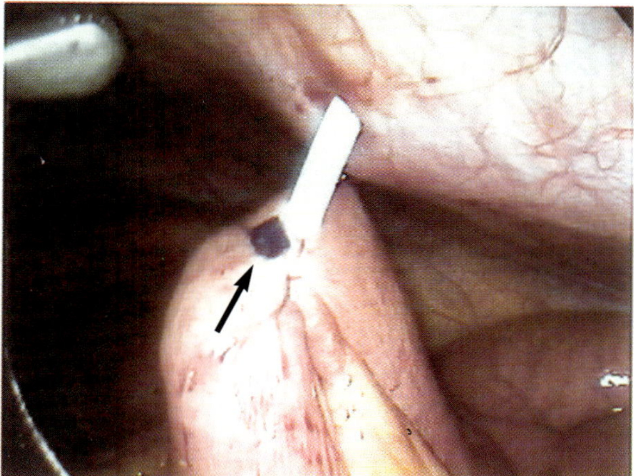

Figure 10.18:   After 2 or 3 running Lembert throws, the suture is ended with a Lapra-Ty suture clip (*arrow*). With the suture clip in place, it secures the suture and the serosal wrap.

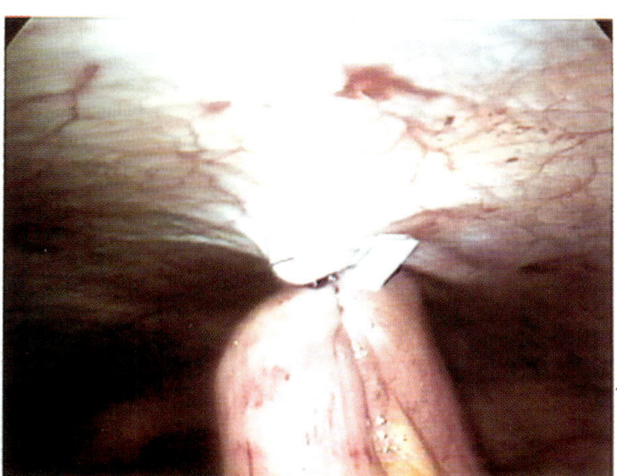

Figure 10.19:   The same stitch as in Figure 10.18, passed through the peritoneum.

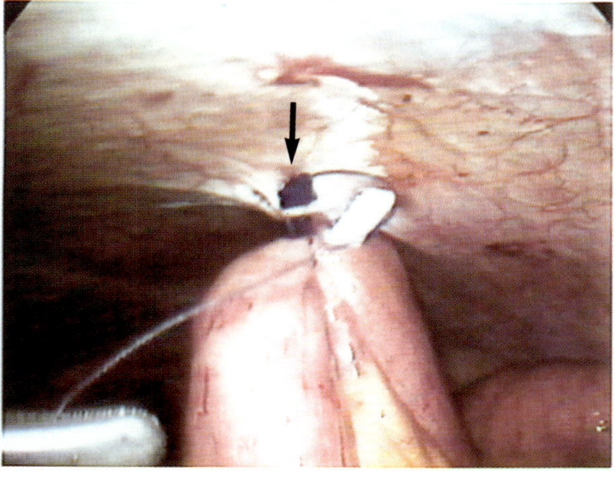

Figure 10.20:   Another Lapra-Ty clip (*arrow*) is placed to secure the stitch to the anterior abdominal wall. The same running stitch is then used to anchor opposite side of the jejunostomy site tube to the anterior abdominal wall.

gastric wall along the greater curvature is anchored to the abdominal wall with the 3–0 Nylon on a Keith needle. The remainder of the procedure is similar to the jejunostomy tube placement.

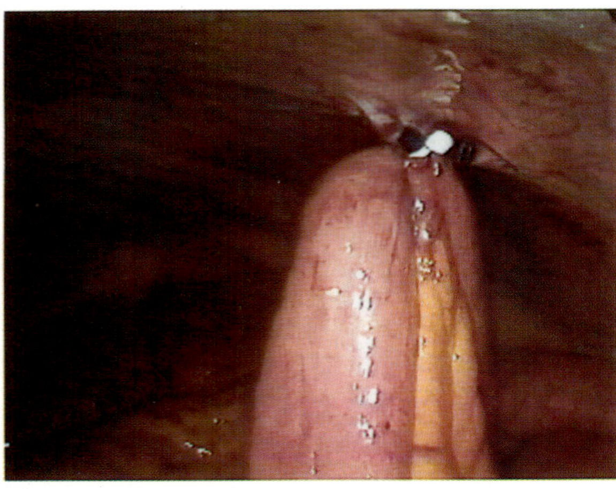

Figure 10.21: The final Lapra-Ty in place. The suture is cut and the needle is removed from the abdominal cavity. The procedure is now complete.

Results

The experience with the laparoscopic-assisted feeding jejunostomy tube placement procedure utilizing the exteriorization technique was successful. There were 17 consecutive patients who had a laparoscopic-assisted feeding jejunostomy using the exteriorization technique. External access was needed as an adjunct to preoperative chemotherapy and/or radiation therapy in 14 patients and for palliation in three patients. There was no associated operative morbidity or mortality. The mean operative time was 100 min (range 36–125 min). Tube feedings were initiated within 24 hours and all patients were advanced to their desired tube-feeding rate without difficulty.

The intracorporeal suturing technique for inserting the feeding jejunostomy tube has been attempted in 15 patients. All patients had their feeding tubes placed by this method and there were no complications related to the procedure. Thirteen patients underwent the procedure and were discharged from the recovery room. The first attempt required 120 minutes but the sixth case took only 49 minutes (Figure 10.22).

Discussion

The laparoscopic approach to enteral feeding tube placement represents a practical application of minimal access surgery. The procedures described in this chapter duplicate the open laparotomy Witzel technique but use the laparoscope to locate the proximal jejunum and even suture the tube in place[9,10]. Other laparoscopic jejunostomy tube procedures which do not require a serosal wrap have been described[11–13]. The needle jejunostomy feeding tubes are 7- to 10-Fr in diameter and are placed in the proximal jejunum using an over-the-wire technique. The jejunostomy tube site is anchored to the abdominal wall with T-fasteners (see Figure 10.4) described by Duh and Way[14]. These fasteners do not require intracorporeal suturing, and they leave skin bolsters on the outside. There are some disadvantages with small-diameter

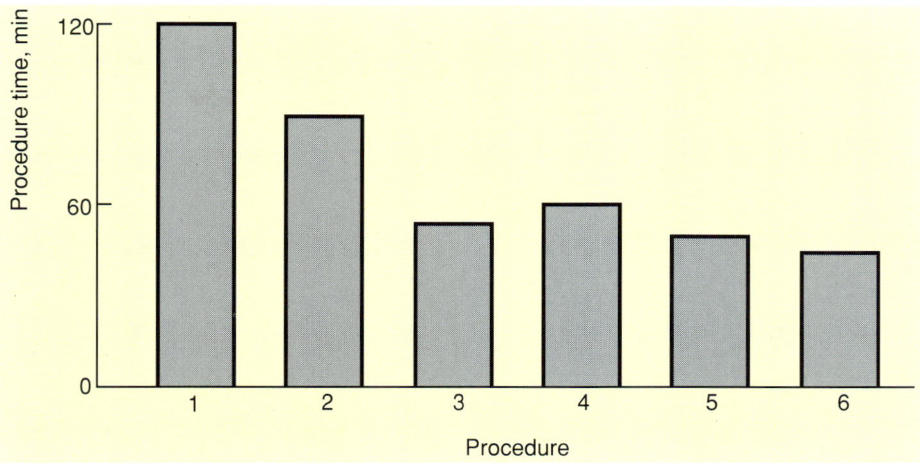

Figure 10.22: Procedure time for the first six laparoscopic-assisted feeding jejunostomy tube placements performed by the senior author.

feeding tubes, however; because of the small bore, elemental feeding solutions are necessary and are three or four times more expensive than the intact protein formulas. The needle jejunostomy tubes can also clog after several weeks of use. Another limitation is that crushed medications cannot be given through these tubes. Lastly, the rationale for the Witzel tunnel is to seal the tube track once the feeding tube is removed. While 7- to 10-Fr tubes are unlikely to create a fistula, a 12-or 14-Fr tube leaves a considerable opening and increases the risk of a fistula when the serosal wrap is not done.

A more significant controversy is the laparoscopic-assisted extracorporeal suturing method vs the intracorporeal suturing procedure. The extracorporeal procedure can be done through a 2–4 cm incision which results in moderate postoperative incisional pain. The advantage of the intracorporeal suturing technique is that it is done solely through 10 mm or less port sites. The disadvantage is that it involves intracorporeal suturing and knot tying. While laparoscopic suturing is difficult, it has become an established part of the laparoscopic Nissen fundoplication. Furthermore, there are two aspects of this procedure that significantly facilitate suturing. One is that the surgeon, the point of suturing and the video monitor should all be aligned, to the surgeon's arms and face in the most comfortable position. The other point is to pin the bowel to the anterior abdominal wall. This takes advantage of the pneumoperitoneum and immobilizes the small bowel so that the surgeon and camera operator are not constantly searching for the jejunostomy site. It also eliminates the need for a fourth port site to grasp the jejunum.

Enteral feeding tubes should only be placed when endoscopic or fluoroscopic placement is not possible. Also, if aspiration is likely with a gastrostomy tube such as in a head-injured patient, a jejunal feeding tube is a reasonable consideration[15,16]. Patients who have upper gastrointestinal malignant disease and require nutritional support to complete either chemotherapy or radiotherapy are candidates for laparoscopic feeding tube placement.

Laparoscopy is greatly expanding beyond the limits of cholecystectomy and Nissen fundoplication. As intracorporeal laparoscopic suturing becomes more common, this procedure will gain acceptance. Training will greatly facilitate laparoscopic suturing and virtual reality simulators will soon be available to assist practicing surgeons and trainees in acquiring this skill.

Acknowledgement

The authors greatly acknowledge the assistance of Mrs Karen Geren in the preparation of this manuscript.

References

1   Jarnagin WR *et al.* (1992) The efficacy and limitations of percutaneous endoscopic gastrostomy. *Arch Surg.* **127**: 261–4.

2   Rosenblum J *et al.* (1990) A new technique for direct percutaneous jejunostomy tube placement. *Am J Gastroent.* **85**: 1165–7.

3   Shike M *et al.* (1991) Direct percutaneous endoscopic jejunostomies, *Gastrointest Endosc.* **37**: 62–5.

4   Ajani JA *et al.* (1993) Preoperative and postoperative combination chemotherapy for potentially resectable gastric carcinoma. *J Nat Cancer Inst.* **85**: 1839–44.

5   Evans DB *et al.* (1991) Adenocarcinoma of the pancreas: Current management of resectable and locally advanced disease. *South Med J.* **84**: 566–70.

6   Douglass HO (1993) Current approaches to multimodality management of advanced pancreatic cancer. *Hepatogastroenterol.* **40**: 433–42.

7   Delcastillo CF and Warshaw L (1993) Peritoneal metastases in pancreatic carcinoma. *Hepatogastroenterol* **40**: 430–2.

8   Fabian TC *et al.* (1993) A prospective analysis of diagnostic laparoscopy in trauma. *Ann Surg.* **217**: 557–65.

9   Ellis LM *et al.* (1992) Laparoscopic feeding jejunostomy tube in oncology patients. *Surg Oncol.* **1**: 245–9.

10   Morris JB *et al.* (1992) Laparoscopic-guided jejunostomy. *Surgery.* **112**: 96–9.

11   O'Regan PJ and Scarrow GD (1990) Laparoscopic jejunostomy. *Endosc.* **22**: 39–40.

12 Reed DN (1992) Percutaneous peritoneoscopic jejunostomy. *Surg Gyn Obstet.* **174**: 527–9.

13 Eltringham WK *et al.* (1993) A laparoscopic technique for full thickness intestinal biopsy and feeding jejunostomy. *Gut.* **34**: 122–4.

14 Duh QY and Way LW (1993) Laparoscopic jejunostomy using T-fasteners as retractors and anchors. *Arch Surg.* **128**: 105–8.

15 Al-Shehri M *et al.* (1990) Feeding jejunostomy: a safe adjunct to laparotomy. *Canc Ass Gen Surg.* **33**: 181–4.

16 Weltz CR *et al.* (1992) Surgical jejunostomy in aspiration risk patients. *Ann Surg.* **215**: 140–5.

11

Thoracoscopic evaluation and resection in pulmonary malignancy

MICHAEL J MACK, STEPHEN R HAZELRIGG and
RODNEY J LANDRENEAU

Introduction

Since the introduction of video thoracoscopy in 1990, it has had an impact on all areas of management of pulmonary malignancy[1]. Thoracoscopy or video-assisted thoracic surgery (VATS) has quickly assumed an important role in the diagnosis and evaluation of pulmonary malignancy, including staging and resective therapy for lung cancer, as well as for the management of the complications of this disease[2]. In this chapter we discuss the role of thoracoscopy in the management of the indeterminate solitary pulmonary nodule, as well as the technique of non-anatomic wedge resection for pulmonary nodules. We then discuss the staging of lung cancer by VATS followed by the definitive resective therapy of lung cancer including VATS lobectomy. Finally we address the role of thoracoscopy in the management of pulmonary metastases and malignant pleural effusions.

The indeterminate solitary pulmonary nodule

Management

Traditional modalities for obtaining a diagnosis of the indeterminate solitary pulmonary nodule include chest X-ray, computerized tomography (CT) fiberoptic bronchoscopy, sputum cytology, fine needle aspiration biopsy, thoracotomy and thoracoscopy[3-8]. The shortcoming with all of these approaches (except thoracotomy) is that it does not allow us to make a definitive diagnosis in a significant percentage of patients, especially those with small nodules or benign disease. This can lead to a false-negative result and may cause an error in management. The advantage of thoracoscopy is its ability to yield a definite diagnosis in virtually every nodule, while avoiding some of the morbidity of an open thoracotomy[9]. However, should all nodules be approached by thoracoscopy?

There are approximately 150,000 new pulmonary nodules discovered annually in the USA[7]. About half of these nodules are malignant, either primary lung cancers or metastases to the lung from other primary tumors. Standard management of indeterminate nodules mandates surgical removal unless benignancy can clearly be demonstrated. If a nodule has been present for two years with no change in size or configuration, it can confidently be declared to be benign[3]. Similarly, if characteristic calcification patterns exist in the nodule, observation of a presumed benign nodule is appropriate. In addition, if the patient is less than 30–35 years of age and no prior history of malignancy exists, the risk of malignancy is less than 1% and no further investigation is necessary[10].

Sputum cytology has a very low yield (15–19% when malignancy exists) and therefore is not appropriate in the diagnostic investigation of indeterminate nodules[11]. Diagnostic bronchoscopy has a similarly low yield in peripheral lung nodules[5] and should play no role in management.

Transthoracic needle aspiration biopsy (TNAB) has been a standard diagnostic technique for lung nodules. However, the only diagnostic result of TNAB that would obviate surgical removal is a specific benign diagnosis. In a review of multiple series of TNAB for solitary nodule diagnosis, the false-negative rate in the presence of malignancy ranged from 3% to 11%[4,12]. When the nodule is 2 cm or smaller, the false-negative rate in malignancy is 40%[13]. There is also a false-positive rate of 1.5–3%[4,12]. Moreover, there is a significant rate of failure to obtain a specific benign diagnosis in confirmed benign disease. In two large series, a specific benign diagnosis was obtained in only 4% and 14% of all patients[14,15], and therefore, these were the only patients who avoided a thoracotomy.

It is against this background of diagnostic options that thoracoscopy should be evaluated. Like thoracotomy, it is virtually 100% accurate diagnostically[9], yet morbidity with this technique is lower than with thoracotomy[16]. In our recent series, and our own subsequent experience, thoracoscopy has accurately and specifically determined the diagnosis in indeterminate nodules. The further benefit of thoracoscopy is that it enables us to treat primary lung cancer during the same procedure that the diagnosis is confirmed. If a malignant diagnosis is obtained, it is possible to stage the pleura and mediastinum and proceed with definitive resective therapy of the tumor.

Candidate nodules for thoracoscopic resection are ≥ 1 cm and located in the outer third of the lung parenchyma (Figure 11.1). Nodules that are smaller than 1 cm or located deeper than 2 cm from a pleural surface are more difficult to locate and resect by thoracoscopic techniques. Nodules less than 1 cm in diameter or located deeper than 2 cm from the pleural surface should undergo preoperative needle localization so that an accurate location can be determined at surgical resection[17] (Figure 11.2).

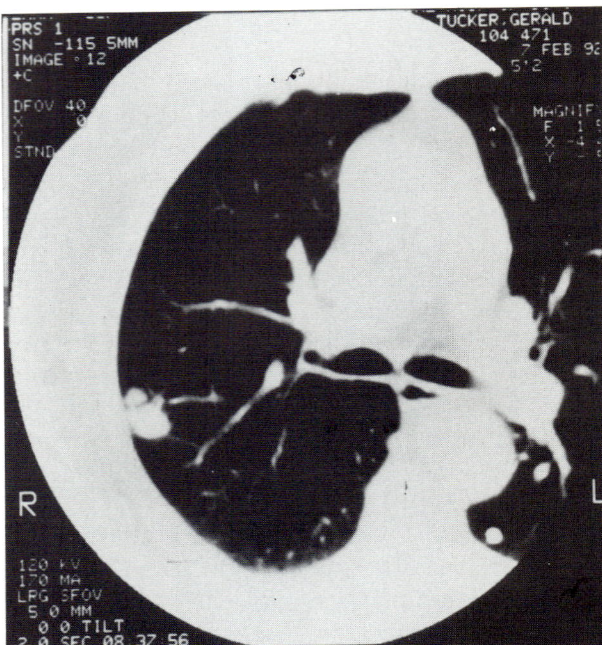

Figure 11.1: Solitary lung nodule that is easily identified and excised by thoracoscopy.

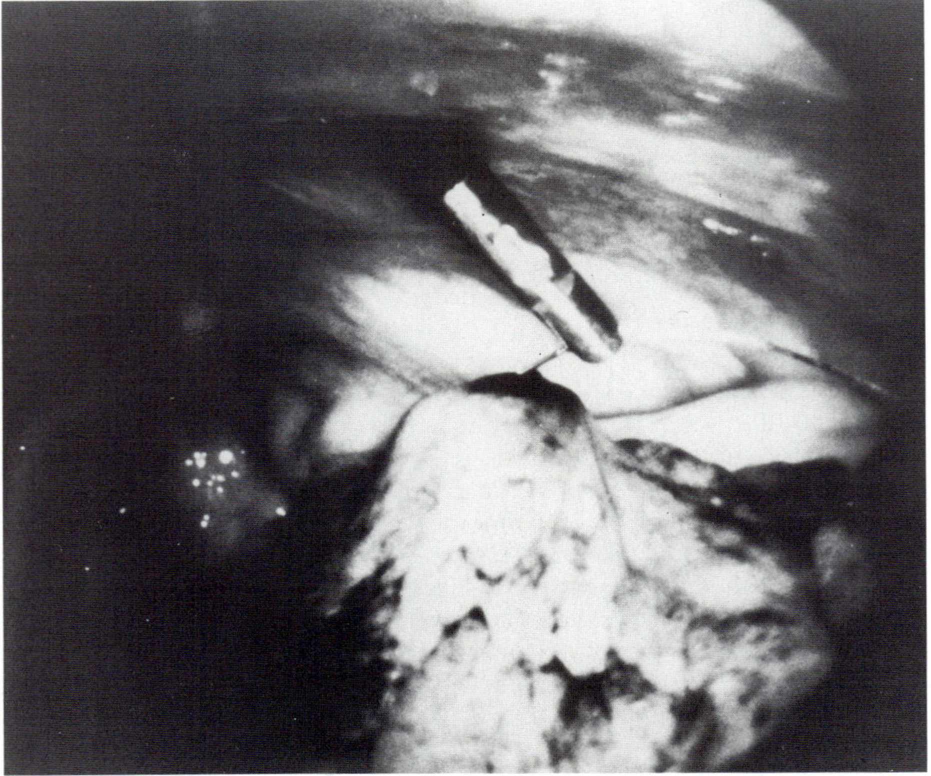

Figure 11.2:   Thoracoscopic view of a localizing wire preoperatively by CT guidance.

Thoracoscopic technique

All procedures are performed under general endotracheal anesthesia with a double lumen tube and with the patient placed in the lateral position[18]. The initial trocar site is usually in the seventh intercostal space in the midaxillary line, but this depends on the location of the nodule. It is often helpful to place one of the trocar sites immediately adjacent to the area of underlying lung suspected to contain the nodule to be resected. This allows a probing digit to be placed through this site, and by digital palpation an occult nodule can be detected beneath the pleural surface (Figure 11.3). The technique of visual inspection combined with digital palpation is sufficient to locate over 90% of nodules. We currently find the needle localization technique to be necessary in less than 10% of patients. The patient's CT scan is always present in the operating room, with frequent re-review necessary intraoperatively to find the location of the nodule accurately.

Once the nodule has been located, lung resection is performed using the endoscopic stapler. We have found the technique (Figure 11.4 a, b and c) to be most helpful. The thoracoscope is placed in the central and inferior portal and

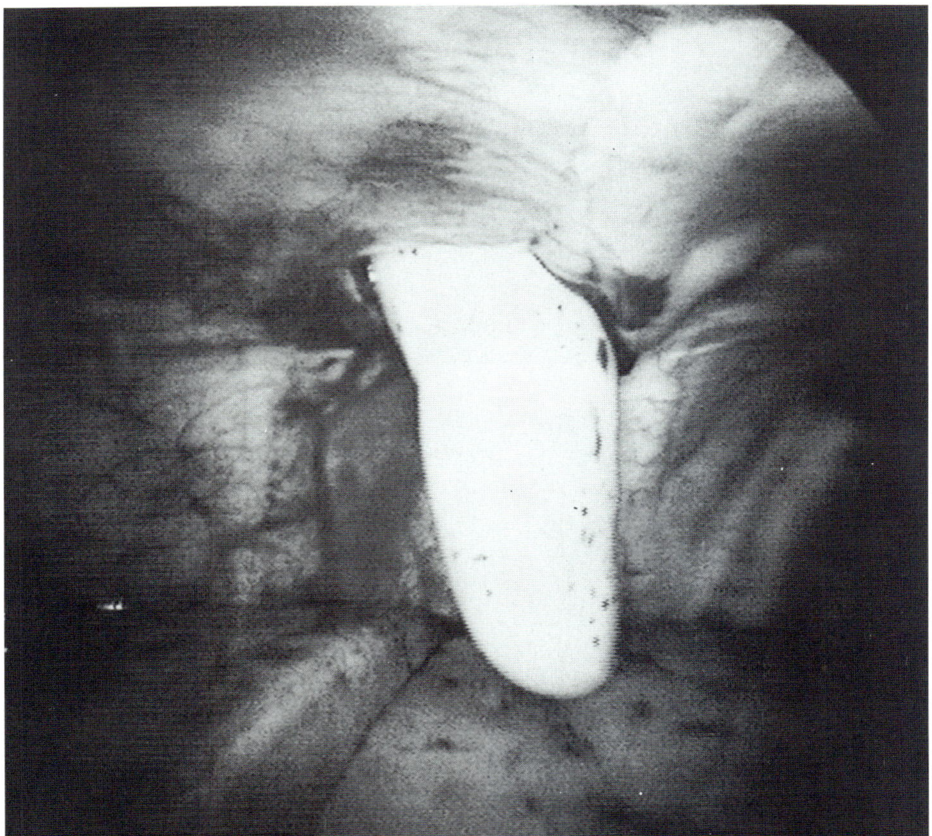

Figure 11.3:   Digit placed through trocar site to palpate the lung to identify a nodule.

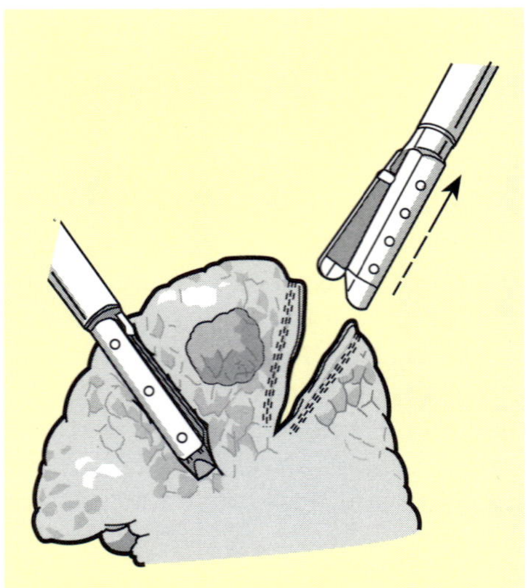

(a)

Figure 11.4: (a) Technique of thoracoscopic lung resection, (b) Initial lung resection with stapler placed from right trocar, (c) Stapler has now been placed from a left trocar site for the second application.

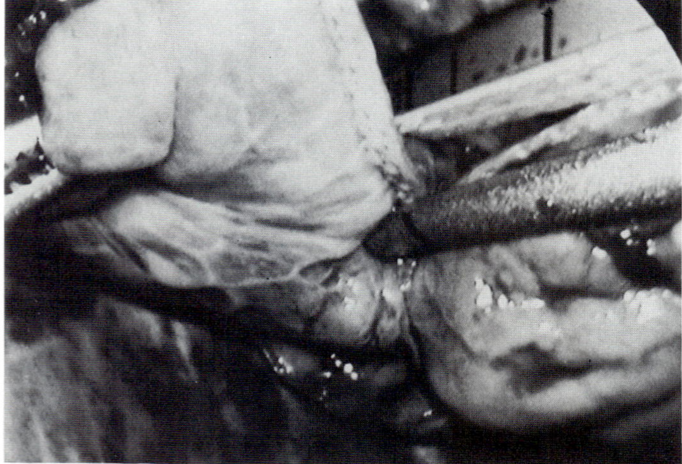

(b)

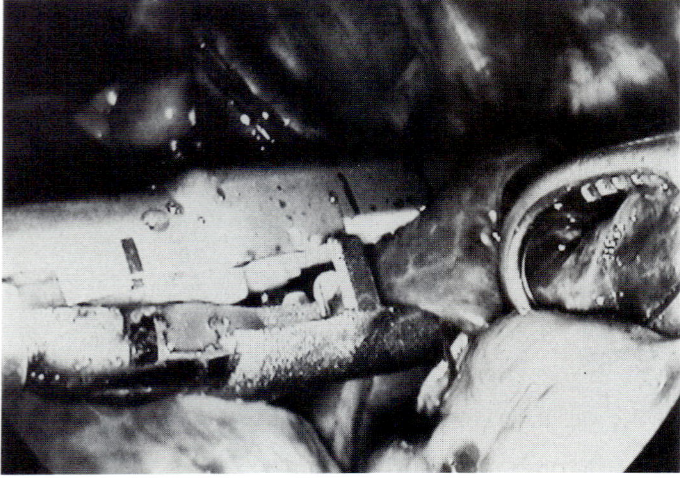

(c)

the two lateral sites are used for the stapler and a grasping instrument. Repeated exchanges of the stapler between the two 'working' ports is the most expeditious method of pulmonary resection. It is usually necessary to reload the stapling instrument three or four times, especially for larger resections. If access through the lateral ports does not allow the appropriate angle for stapler application, the scope is moved to one of the lateral ports and the stapling instrument is placed through the central portal. By this repeated exchange process, almost all nodules that have been appropriately selected as outlined above can be resected using the endoscopic stapler. The next generation of endoscopic stapling instruments will have jaws that can be angulated up to 60°. This articulation of the instrument will greatly simplify the process of stapler application at the appropriate angle on the lung.

Significant experience has been gained with use of the Nd:YAG laser for endoscopic pulmonary resection[19] (Figure 11.5). This process is rather cumbersome, slow and difficult to master, and therefore we rarely use the laser for nodule resection.

Once a nodule has been resected, it is placed in a specimen bag (Figure 11.6) for removal through a trocar site if there is any suspicion of malignancy. Tumor seeding of trocar sites from unprotected removal of malignant specimens has been reported to the VATS Registry[20]. If the nodule is small and totally surrounded by lung parenchyma, placement in a specimen bag for removal may not be necessary.

Once a frozen section diagnosis has been obtained on the indeterminate nodule, and if it is appropriate to proceed with further lung resection (see below), a lobectomy is then performed by either open or VATS techniques. If the nodule is benign, or if a wedge resection with appropriate margins is the limit of the planned resection, the staple lines are checked for pneumostasis and hemostasis, the lung is reinflated and a small chest tube (20 Fr) is placed through an anterior trocar site. Intensive postoperative care is seldom necessary and the chest tube is removed as soon as it is ascertained that there is no air

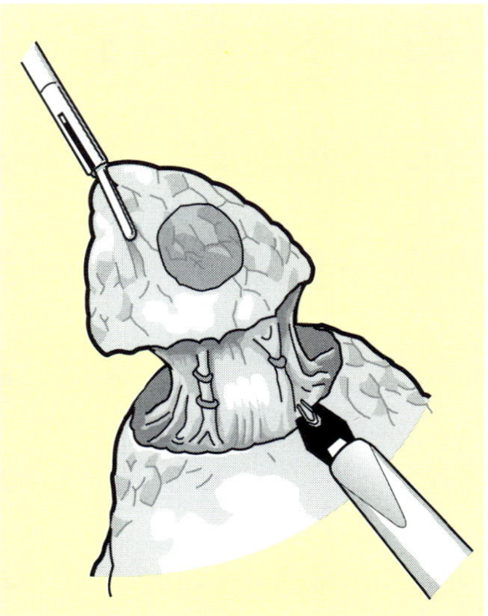

Figure 11.5:　Technique of laser lung resection for a pulmonary nodule.

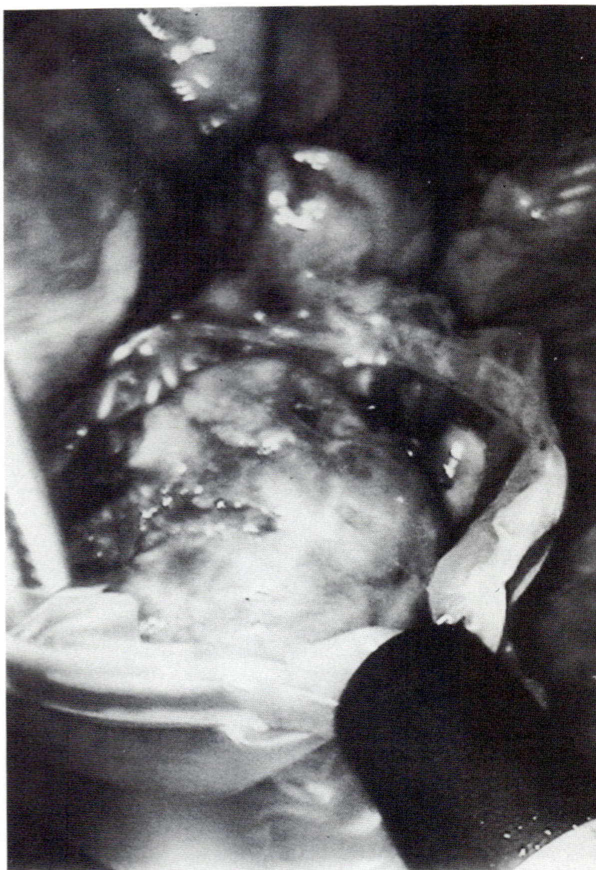

Figure 11.6: Resected lung specimen containing a malignancy being placed in a specimen sac for extraction to prevent chest-wall seeding.

leak, which is frequently in the recovery room. The chest tube is the major cause of postoperative pain, so using a small tube and removing it promptly lessens pain and shortens the hospital stay.

Staging of pulmonary malignancy

Preoperative stay

Staging of pulmonary malignancy is performed both preoperatively and intraoperatively. Appropriate preoperative staging should include CT to assess the hilar and mediastinal lymph node-bearing areas. There is controversy about whether a CT scan is sufficient for preoperative staging or whether a cervical mediastinal exploration (CME) is necessary for all candidates. The false-negative rate of CT scans is reported to be approximately 15% for nodes less than 1 cm in the mediastinum[21]. However, this false-negative rate is significantly lower if no nodes are present on the scan. It is our present practice to perform a CME only if lymphadenopathy is present in the mediastinum on CT scan.

Cervical mediastinal exploration

When performing cervical mediastinal exploration, we are currently evaluating the technique of video mediastinoscopy (Figure 11.7). This is performed by a simple modification of the standard mediastinoscope, with an additional channel for the placement of a 5 mm telescope with video camera attached. The benefits of this technique appear to be better visualization (and therefore evaluation) of the mediastinal lymph node-bearing areas. The subazygous nodes (level 4R) and subcarinal nodes (level 7) appear to be more readily accessed by the video techniques. It may be more accurate in determining intranodal vs extranodal spread of tumor, and also seems to make it easier to teach the technique to thoracic surgical trainees.

Thoracoscopy

For staging of left-sided malignancy, we no longer employ a second left interspace exploration (Chamberlain procedure). Instead we use left thoracoscopy to evaluate the aortopulmonary window[13]. In our experience, thoracoscopy affords better visualization and therefore more accurate staging of not only the anterior mediastinum and cardiopulmonary window (levels 5 and 6) but also the inferior pulmonary ligament (level 8), compared with the Chamberlain procedure[22].

The technique is illustrated in Figure 11.8. Generous sampling of these lymph nodes can be performed by this technique prior to definitive resective therapy.

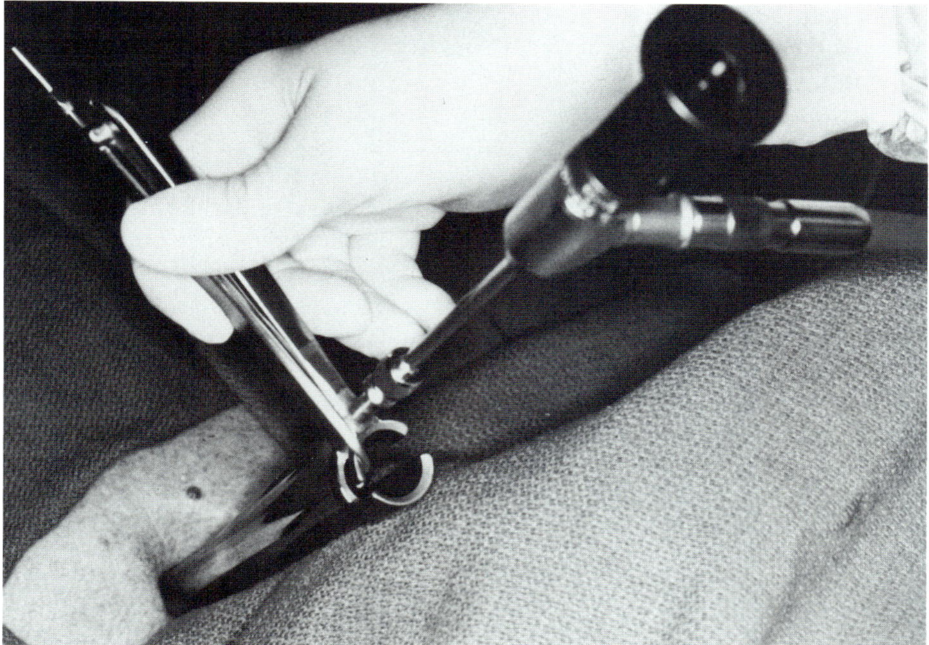

Figure 11.7:   Mediastinoscope with video attachment in place for mediastinal exploration.

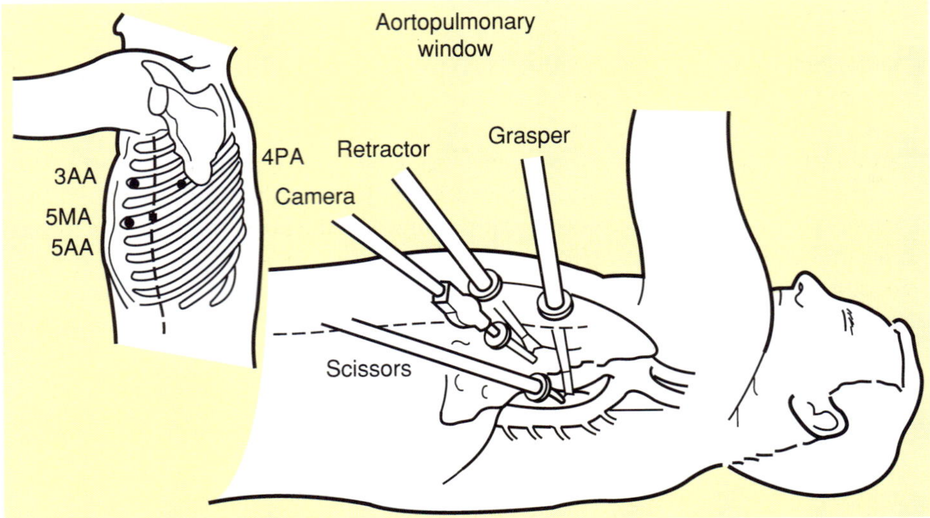

Figure 11.8:   Thoracoscopic technique of biopsy of aortopulmonary window lymph nodes.

Intraoperative staging

Complete intraoperative staging before anticipated lung resection for pulmonary malignancy includes complete thoracoscopic examination of the chest cavity for evidence of pleural, parenchymal or regional nodal metastases. During the past two years, we have discovered unsuspected pleural metastases on four occasions during thoracotomy for lobectomy (Figure 11.9). It has therefore become our practice to perform exploratory thoracoscopy prior to a planned procedure, to avoid a needless thoracotomy in an unresectable patient.

The technique is relatively straightforward. An initial trocar is placed in the seventh intercostal space in the midaxillary line and used for placement of the thoracoscope. An additional site is placed in the sixth intercostal space in the anterior axillary line and used for a lung-grasping instrument. These two sites are used for chest tube placement at the conclusion of the procedure. Exploration of all visceral and parietal pleural surfaces is performed including the fissures and diaphragmatic surfaces. Any suspicious lesions are biopsied and sent for frozen section analysis. Close examination of the preoperative CT scan occasionally reveals suspicious areas of pleural thickening or puckering. However, we have encountered pleural involvement with tumor without prior CT scan evidence, even in retrospect.

Once total examination of all pleural surfaces is complete, the regional lymph node-bearing areas are examined and sampled as outlined above. If our staging reveals no evidence of tumor spread, definitive resective therapy is then undertaken.

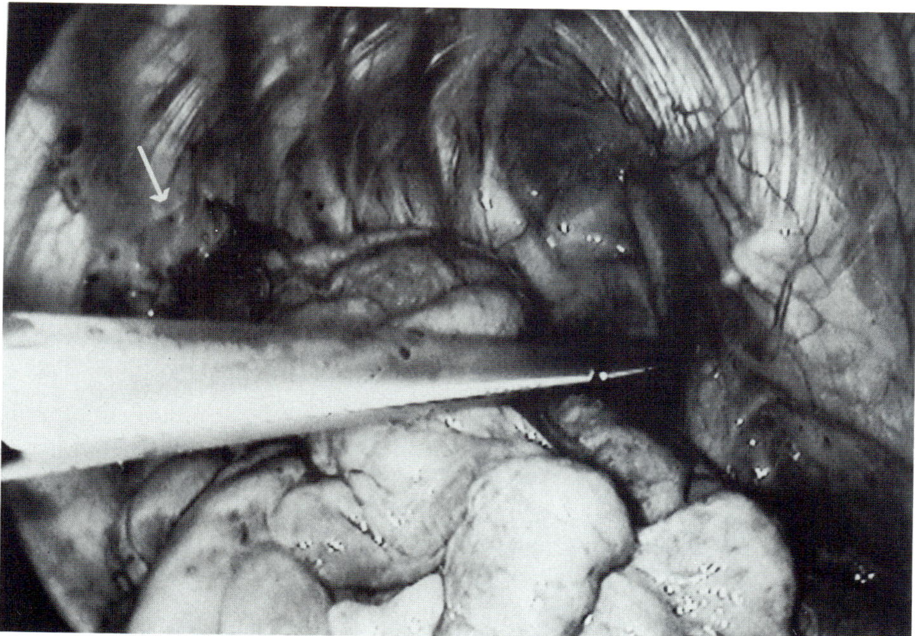

Figure 11.9:   Unsuspected pleural metastasis (*arrow*) discovered at time of thoracotomy for lung resection.

Resective therapy for lung cancer

Definitive resection for lung cancer is by either localized resection or formal lobectomy. Both methods of resection can be performed by either open or thoracoscopic techniques.

Wedge resection

Local wedge resection as definitive therapy for lung cancer performed by thoracoscopy has been described by Shennib[23]. Thoracoscopic wedge resection for primary lung malignancy is appropriate therapy in patients with limited pulmonary function or with a compromised general medical condition, old age or frailty, in whom a thoracotomy and lobectomy is not possible. If a wedge resection is the planned operation due to these conditions, then performance by thoracoscopic techniques decreases postoperative pain and morbidity[16].

The technique for wedge resection of primary lung cancer is the same as that described for the indeterminate lung nodule. A clean surgical margin of at least 1 cm around the malignancy should be obtained, although distortion of lung tissue around the nodule by the staple lines may occasionally make this difficult to determine. Again, removal from the chest in a protective endoscopic specimen bag is mandatory.

However, there is controversy about appropriate resection in patients with adequate pulmonary function and whose general medical condition would tolerate a lobectomy. Although data from the Lung Cancer Study Group showed no survival benefit of lobectomy compared with wedge resection in stage I lung cancer[24], there was a higher loco-regional recurrence rate of 22% with local resection vs 8% with lobectomy. It should be emphasized that both procedures were performed by open techniques before the VATS era. Although there is no demonstrated improvement in survival with lobectomy, it remains our preferred operation in patients who can tolerate it.

VATS lobectomy

Numerous investigators have demonstrated the feasibility of performing pulmonary lobectomy by thoracoscopic techniques. Published series of 200 patients have been accumulated without mortality and with minimal morbidity[25,26]. However, inasmuch as the procedure has been demonstrated to be safe in a relatively small number of cases in a few centers, clear-cut benefits have yet to be demonstrated[27].

Patient selection

Most investigators have limited candidates for VATS lobectomy to those with preoperative stage I disease. Tumors should be less than 3 cm in diameter since large tumors make extraction of the specimen from the chest impossible. They should be peripheral in location without extension to the hilum, since dissection of the hilar structures is the limiting step of the procedure. For the same reasons, hilar lymphadenopathy should not be present because of difficulty dissecting the hilar vessels and bronchus.

The best tumors for VATS lobectomy are those in the lower lobes, especially the left lower lobe. Lower lobectomies are technically easier to perform than middle or upper lobectomies and a surgeon's early experience should be limited to the lower lobes. Incomplete fissures prolong the procedure and dissection and completion of the fissures is quite difficult. The surgeon must be prepared to convert to an open procedure if extensive hilar lymphadenopathy or incomplete fissure exist.

Technique

The standard technique for VATS lobectomy requires two incisions of 1 cm each and one 'accessory' or 'utility' incision of 6–7 cm. This longer incision is required for specimen removal at the conclusion of the procedure, but it is made initially to utilize it for access for standard thoracic instrumentation. The two smaller incisions are placed in the seventh intercostal space in the midaxillary and posterior axillary lines. For upper lobectomies, the *posterior* portal is placed in the third or fourth intercostal space *anteriorly* for scope placement and visualization of the superior aspect of the hilum. The accessory incision is made in the fifth intercostal space in the anterior axillary line. Since rib spreading is the major contributor to postoperative pain, it is *not* used since it would negate the benefits of the VATS approach.

Once the incisions have been made and access has been gained to the thoracic cavity, initial exploratory thoracoscopy is performed. During this exploration, pleural metastases are ruled out, the mediastinum is examined, and confirmation of the tumor in the appropriate lobe is obtained. Note is also made of the completeness of the fissures and whether any hilar involvement with tumor extension or lymphadenopathy exists. If the fissures are incomplete or if initial dissection of the hilar structures proves difficult, conversion to an open procedure should now be done.

Dissection is begun in the hilum and attention is directed toward the pulmonary vein first since it is the most accessible structure. If the lower-lobe pulmonary vein is to be divided, the inferior pulmonary ligament is divided using endoscopic scissors with electrocautery attachment. For retraction of the lung, we have found the curved ring forceps to be quite helpful. We may place two or three different instruments, retractors or a scope through the accessory incision simultaneously.

The pulmonary vein is dissected free using a combination of sharp and blunt dissection. We use a tonsil-tip suction device or an endoscopic kittner to free the target vessel from surrounding tissue. Once the vein has been totally mobilized, a right-angled clamp is placed around it to ensure freedom and to create enough space for placement of the jaws of the endoscopic stapler. Placement of a 0 silk suture around the vessel for traction will aid stapler application. The jaws of a vascular endoscopic stapler (2.5 mm staples) are then placed across the vessel. Because the jaws of the stapler do not yet articulate, trials of application from different incisions may be necessary to obtain proper placement. Complete placement of the vessel within the staple line should be verified before firing. The stapler applies three rows of staples on each side and cuts between them. Some concern has arisen about possible stapler malfunction in this relatively uncontrolled surgical setting. If this is a worry, the knife blade can be removed from the stapler before application. This will allow for verification of two complete sets of staple lines before cutting. The vessel can then be divided with the endoscopic scissors.

The next hilar structures to be approached are the interlobar or segmental pulmonary arteries. Again, the vessels are dissected free by a combination of sharp and blunt dissection. Smaller segmental pulmonary arteries can be ligated by a 2–0 silk suture or application of an endoscopic clip (or both). The interlobar artery and larger segmental pulmonary arteries (anterior, apical-posterior trunk) can be best managed by the vascular endoscopic stapler (Figure 11.10). The exception to this technique of dividing the pulmonary artery next is the left upper lobe, when better access is obtained by dividing the upper-lobe bronchus before the anterior segmental pulmonary artery is controlled.

Once the vascular structures have been ligated and divided, attention is turned to the bronchus. Any surrounding soft tissue is divided by sharp and/or blunt dissection until sufficient visualization and mobilization has occurred for proper stapler placement. Bronchial arteries are ligated with endoscopic clips. A 3.5 mm endoscopic stapler (blue cartridge) is then applied. The lung is

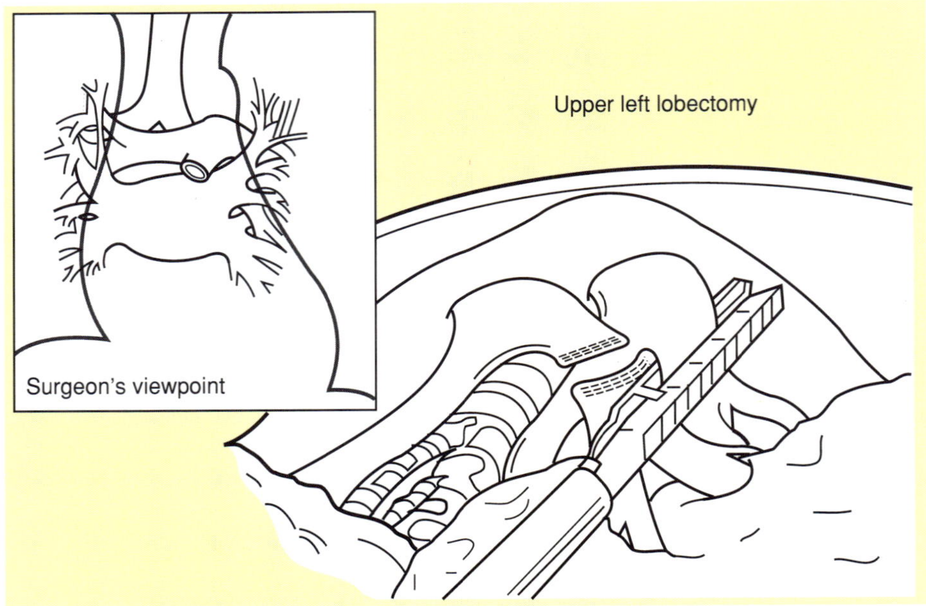

Figure 11.10:   Technique of thoracoscopic left upper lobectomy using the endoscopic stapler to divide the left superior pulmonary vein and the apical–posterior pulmonary artery trunk.

inflated to ensure that compromise of the remaining airway has not occurred, whereupon the stapler is fired.

The specimen is then retrieved from the chest cavity. Constant, gentle traction is used to 'milk' the lobe through the accessory incision (Figure 11.11). Occasionally a retractor is necessary briefly to spread the ribs sufficiently to extract the specimen.

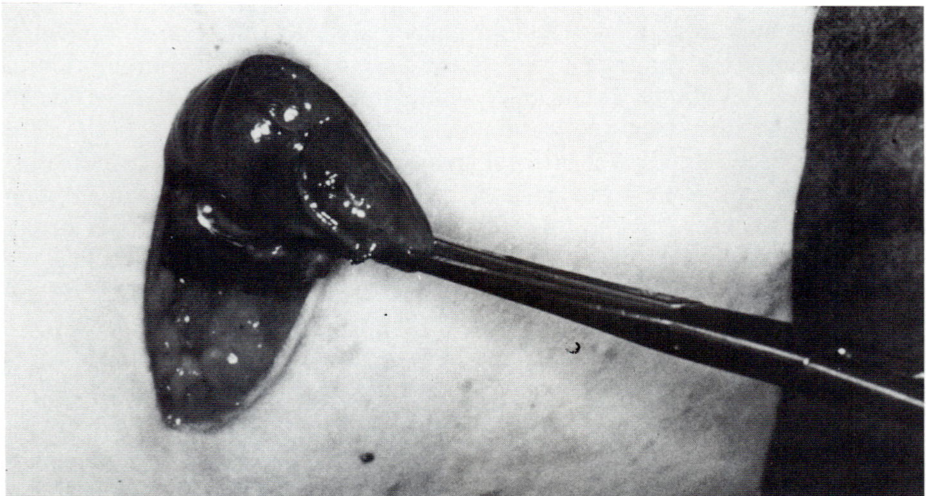

Figure 11.11:   Extraction of a resected lobe through the accessory incision.

Once the specimen has been removed, complete hemostasis obtained and a secure bronchial stump ascertained, the lung is reexpanded. Small chest tubes (20–24 Fr) are placed through the two trocar sites and the accessory incision is sutured. Care in an intensive care unit is generally not necessary and discharge is usually on day three or four after chest tube removal.

Pneumonectomy

VATS pneumonectomy has been successfully performed in a few instances, all on the left side[25,26]. The technique is generally similar to that of a lobectomy, except that of course dissection in the fissure is not necessary. The only variation in technique involves the mainstem bronchus. A 4.8 mm staple is necessary for secure closure of the main bronchus and does not yet exist in an endoscopic stapler. With the specimen in place, however, a standard TA30–4.8 stapler cannot be placed around the bronchus. Therefore, we staple the bronchus more distal to the planned resection line with the 3.5 mm endoscopic stapler, remove the specimen and restaple the bronchus with the TA stapler more proximally.

Conclusions

Although a fair amount of experience with VATS lobectomy has been gained in many centers, no clear benefit has yet been demonstrated. Operative time is approximately 50% longer than by the standard open technique, and the conversion rate for technical difficulty is approximately 25%. A recent randomized study between VATS and open lobectomy[28] showed no clear benefit for the thoracoscopic approach. Morbidity and length of stay were equivalent for both groups.

However, it does appear that an extensive experience is necessary to overcome initial difficulties. After 20 VATS lobectomies and over 500 total thoracoscopic procedures, we are only just beginning to find that the VATS approach has real advantages.

We also routinely now use video assistance for all open procedures. This 'hybrid' procedure or video-assisted thoracotomy appears to allow open procedures to be performed with less rib-spreading, smaller incisions and with better lighting and magnification.

Metastatic pulmonary disease

Thoracoscopy has been used for the management of metastatic nodules in the lung[11]. The technique is quite effective when used as a diagnostic modality in patients with a previous history of malignancy. Its role as a therapeutic procedure in patients with known metastatic tumor burden, however, is somewhat controversial.

Lung nodules in approximately one-third of patients with a previous history of malignancy will prove to be a new primary lung cancer depending upon the site of the original tumor[29]. Often the diagnosis eludes less invasive attempts including needle aspiration biopsy. Metastatic nodules are usually peripheral, frequently in a subpleural location, and therefore lend themselves quite well to thoracoscopic identification and resection. A recent series by Dowling *et al.*[11], in which thoracoscopy was used as primarily a diagnostic modality, yielded a correct diagnosis in all 72 patients.

The role of thoracoscopy as a therapeutic modality is not well defined nor accepted. The inability to normally palpate the whole lung to detect occult metastases not apparent on CT scans has been held as a shortcoming of the procedure. However, a survival benefit has been demonstrated in selected malignancies (soft-tissue sarcoma of the extremity) when occult contralateral tumor has existed[30]. In terms of survival, similarly, the benefits of thoracotomy over median sternotomy (with the ability to palpate both lungs) has not been demonstrated[31]. However, with slip-ring spiral CT scanning giving better definition to the lung, nodules as small as 2 mm can be detected. As this technology becomes more widespread it is anticipated that the role of thoracoscopy will expand as a therapeutic procedure in patients with metastatic lung nodules.

Malignant pleural effusions

Malignant involvement of the pleura from lung cancer or from tumors metastatic to the pleura from another site represents a late stage and often difficult aspect of the disease to manage (Figure 11.12). When conservative measures such as thoracentesis or chest tube drainage have failed to control the locally effusive process, or when the etiology remains unclear despite these less invasive attempts at diagnosis, thoracoscopy presents the optimal form of management[32].

There is quite a high success rate for controlling the effusive process, due to the ability to drain totally the chest cavity under direct vision, break up loculations and evenly distribute a sclerosing agent over all parietal surfaces. It is our present practice to use talc as the sclerosing substance (Figure 11.13) since it is easy to use, effective and inexpensive[23]. The procedures is performed with two trocar sites, or only one if an operating thoracoscope is available. Our success rate exceeds 95%, the only failures occurring when there is inability to reexpand the lung due to tumor entrapment. In this instance, a pleural-peritoneal shunt represents the only method of palliation.

Conclusion

Thoracoscopy has rapidly evolved from a rarely applied diagnostic procedure for pleural disease to a widely utilized procedure to manage many aspects of pulmonary malignancy. There is an ever-expanding role for thoracoscopy as a diagnostic procedure for the indeterminate solitary pulmonary nodule, gradually replacing other diagnostic modalities. It has high diagnostic accuracy and

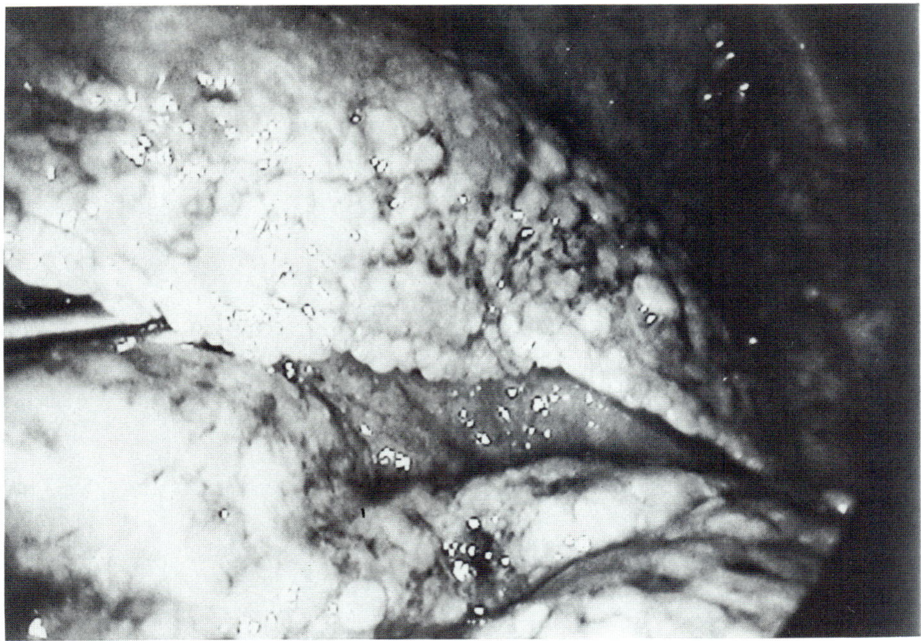

Figure 11.12:   Extensive pleural involvement with metastatic adenocarcinoma of the lung.

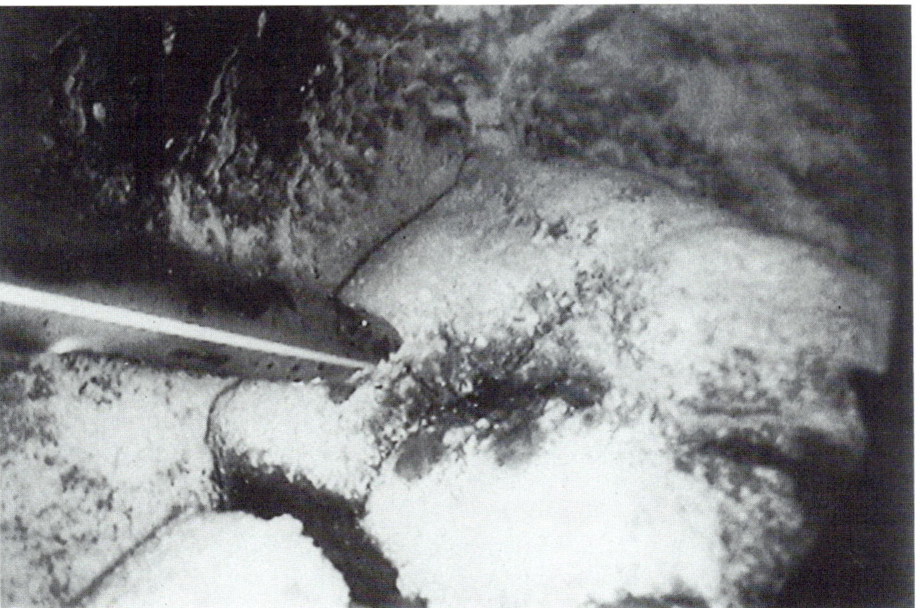

Figure 11.13:   Talc has been insufflated into the chest covering all pleural surfaces.

allows the surgeon to proceed immediately to a more definitive procedure at the same sitting.

There is also a significant role in the staging of lung cancer. Although we still employ cervical mediastinal exploration for the staging of right-sided tumors, we have extended it by the use of video-mediastinoscopy. Left thoracoscopy has replaced the Chamberlain procedure in our practice for the staging of the aortopulmonary window and left-sided tumors.

As definitive resective therapy for lung cancer in patients with poor pulmonary reserve or compromised general medical condition, thoracoscopy is a less invasive technique for localized lung-sparing wedge resections. However, its role in patients who can otherwise tolerate a lobectomy is controversial because it does not offer increased chances of survival.

Although the experience with VATS lobectomy is rapidly increasing, clear-cut benefits of the technique over a muscle-sparing thoracotomy—especially when epidural analgesia is used for postoperative pain management—have not been defined. The procedure is still quite complex and awaits advances in surgical instrumentation, including articulating staplers.

There is a definite role for thoracoscopy as a diagnostic modality for metastatic disease when less invasive attempts at diagnosis have failed. However, its role as a therapeutic procedure is not clear. Improved accuracy of spiral CT scanning may define a greater role for thoracoscopy.

Finally, thoracoscopy is a highly effective method of controlling some of the complications of lung cancer, including malignant pleural effusions, by talc pleurodesis.

Thoracoscopy has made a significant impact on the management of intrathoracic neoplastic processes in a short time. Its role is likely to grow as surgeons become more experienced, as instrumentation becomes more surgeon-friendly and as treatment modalities change. With an anticipated role for gene therapy in lung cancer in the near future, thoracoscopy will present the least invasive approach for harvesting tumor.

References

1 Landreneau RJ *et al.* (1993) The role of thoracoscopy in the management of intrathoracic neoplastic processes. *Sem Thor Cardiovasc Surg.* **5**: 219–28.

2 Landreneau RJ *et al.* (1992) Thoracoscopy for the diagnosis and treatment of intrathoracic malignancy. *Proc Am Soc Clin Onc.* **11**: 291.

3 Steele JD and Buell P (1973) Asymptomatic solitary pulmonary nodules, host survival, tumor size, and growth rates. *J Thor Cardiovasc Surg.* **65**: 140–51.

4 Westcott JL (1980) Direct percutaneous needle aspiration of localized pulmonary lesions: results in 422 patients. *Radiol.* **137**: 31–5.

5 Fletcher EC and Levin DC (1982) Flexible fiberoptic bronchoscopy and fluoroscopically guided transbronchial biopsy in the management of solitary pulmonary nodules. *Western J Med.* **136**: 477–83.

6   Levine MS *et al.* (1988) Transthoracic needle aspiration biopsy following negative fiberoptic bronchoscopy in solitary pulmonary nodules. *Chest.* **93**: 1152–5.

7   Lillington GA (1991) Management of solitary pulmonary nodules. *Dis Month.* **37**: 271–318.

8   Mack MJ *et al.* (1993) Present role of thoracoscopy in the diagnosis and treatment of diseases of the chest. *Ann Thor Surg.* **54**: 403–9.

9   Mack MJ *et al.* (1993) Thoracoscopy for the diagnosis of the indeterminate solitary pulmonary nodule. *Ann Thor Surg.* **56**: 825–32.

10   Midthun DE *et al.* (1992) Clinical strategies for solitary pulmonary nodule. *Ann Rev Med.* **54**: 195–208.

11   Dowling RD *et al.* (1993) Video-assisted thoracoscopic resection of pulmonary metastases. *Ann Thor Surg.* **56**: 772–5.

12   Khouri NF *et al.* (1986) Transthoracic needle aspiration biopsy of benign and malignant lung lesions. *Am J Roentg.* **144**: 281–8.

13   Berquist TH *et al.* (1980) Transthoracic needle biopsy accuracy and complications in relation to location and type of lesion. *Mayo Clin Proc.* **55**: 475–81.

14   Calhoun P *et al.* (1986) The clinical outcome of needle aspirations of the lung when cancer is not diagnosed. *Ann Thor Surg.* **41**: 592–6.

15   Khouri NF *et al.* (1987) The solitary pulmonary nodule: assessment, diagnosis and management. *Chest.* **91**: 128–33.

16   Landreneau RJ *et al.* (1993) Postoperative pain-related morbidity: video-assisted thoracic surgery versus thoracotomy. *Ann Thor Surg.* **56**: 1285–9.

17   Mack MJ *et al.* (1993) Techniques for localization of pulmonary nodules for thoracoscopic resection *J Thor Cardiovasc Surg.* **106**: 550–3.

18   Landreneau RJ *et al.* (1992) Video assisted thoracic surgery: basic technical concepts and intercostal approach strategies. *Ann Thor Surg.* **54**: 800–7.

19   Landreneau RJ *et al.* (1991) Nd:YAG laser assisted pulmonary resections. *Ann Thor Surg.* **51**: 973–8.

20   Hazelrigg SR *et al.* (1993) Video assisted thoracic surgery study group data. *Ann Thor Surg.* **45**: 1039–44.

21   Hazelrigg SR *et al.* (1993) Video assisted thoracic surgery for mediastinal disease. *Chest Surg Clin N Am.* **3**: 283–97.

22 Landreneau RJ *et al.* (1993) Thoracoscopic mediastinal lymph node sampling: a useful approach to mediastinal lymph node stations inaccesible to cervical mediastinoscopy. *J Thor Cardiovasc Surg.* **105**: 554–8.

23 Shennib H *et al.* (1993) Video assisted thoracoscopic wedge resection of T1 lung cancer in high risk patients. *Ann Thor Surg.* **218**: 555–60.

24 Ginsberg RJ and Rubenstein LV (1991) Patients with T1N0 non-small cell lung cancer. *Lung Cancer.* **7**: 83.

25 Kirby TJ *et al.* (1993) Initial experience with video-assisted thoracoscopic lobectomy. *Ann Thor Surg.* **56**: 1248–53.

26 Roviaro G *et al.* (1993) Major pulmonary resections: pneumonectomies and lobectomies. *Ann Thor Surg.* **56**: 779–83.

27 Kirby TJ and Rice TW (1993) Thoracoscopic lobectomy. *Ann Thor Surg.* **56**: 784–6.

28 Kirby TJ *et al.* (1994) A randomized comparison of thoracoscopy versus open thoracotomy for stage I lung cancer. *J Thor Cardiovasc Surg.* In press.

29 Roth JA (1989) Treatment of metastatic cancer to lung. In: De Vita VT, Hellman S, Rosenberg SA (eds): *Cancer: Principles and Practice of Oncology*, Lippincott, Philadelphia. pp. 2261–75.

30 Putnam JB *et al.* (1984) Analysis of prognostic factors in patients undergoing resection of pulmonary metastases from soft tissue sarcoma. *J Thor Cardiovasc Surg.* **87**: 260–7.

31 Roth JA *et al.* (1986) Comparison of median sternotomy and thoracoscopy for resection of pulmonary metastases in patients with soft tissue sarcoma. *Ann Thor Surg.* **42**: 143–8.

32 LoCicero J III (1993) Thoracoscopic management of malignant pleural effusion. *Ann Thor Surg.* **56**: 641–3.

33 Bresticker MA *et al.* (1993) Optimal pleurodesis: a comparison study. *Ann Thor Surg.* **55**: 364–7.

12

Laparoscopic approach for regional hepatic chemotherapy in the treatment of primary or metastatic malignancy

MORRIS E FRANKLIN JR, RICHARD F NOREM and
RICHARD STUBBS

Introduction

The management of hepatic malignancy, whether primary or metastatic, is a serious challenge for physicians. Currently a variety of modalities are advocated, including regional arterial infusion of chemotherapeutic medications. The rationale behind intra-arterial chemotherapy has been well established, and there is much evidence for its beneficial effects. On the other hand, percutaneous routes of treatment have limited life-expectancy and are somewhat unpredictable and unreliable. Unfortunately open surgical placement of hepatic artery catheters and infusion devices carries an established morbidity and mortality of up to 25% in these already debilitated patients[1–5]. Laparoscopy has opened up new opportunities for treatment by allowing direct access to the hepatic arterial system and placement of a permanent in-dwelling catheter without the need for a formal laparotomy.

Case report

Our first experience with this minimal access approach was in August 1993. A 51-year-old black male was admitted to our hospital with a large, non-obstructing, unresectable adenocarcinoma of the rectum which encased the pelvic vasculature. The initial investigation revealed pre-encephalopathy and a large number of liver metastases. After careful consideration and consultation with the patient and his family, as well as all the practitioners involved, we decided to treat the patient initially with regional chemotherapy via hepatic arterial catheterization with a permanent infusion device. An arteriogram was performed to determine the exact arterial supply to the liver, as well as to define any congenital anomalies.

The procedure was performed under general anesthesia, using a nasogastric tube and urinary catheter. Six × 10 mm trocar/cannulas were placed as shown in Figure 12.1:

- in the supra-umbilical midline

- just to the right and just to the left of midline in the epigastrium

- in the mid-right and in the mid-left lateral abdomen

- in the left upper quadrant (Figure 1).

As the patient was in the reverse Trendelenberg position the liver was gently retracted anteriorly with a non-traumatic fan retractor. The antrum of the stomach was gently retracted caudally. Gentle dissection was undertaken at the gastrohepatic ligament to identify the common hepatic, gastroduodenal and proper hepatic arteries. Care was taken to identify and ligate the small veins and lymphatics in this area.

Tissue in this area may be somewhat thickened depending on the amount of portal vascular and lymphatic flow resistance. In this case, having isolated the main arteries, we clipped the distally visualized gastroduodenal artery while double-looping a silk tie around the proximal portion of the vessel, to provide physical countertraction, act as a tourniquet, and finally to anchor the inserted catheter at the conclusion of the procedure. Laparoscopic vascular bulldog clamps were applied to the most proximal visualized portion of the common hepatic artery and the most distal visualized portion of the proper hepatic artery (Figure 12.2). The laparoscopic bulldog clamps provided:

- vascular control

- haemostasis during the arteriotomy, while leaving all laparoscopic cannulas open for other instruments to be inserted

- ease of application and removal.

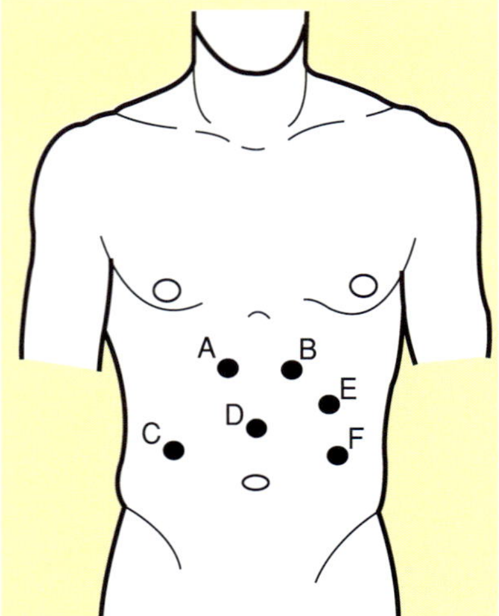

Figure 12.1: Trocar/cannula placement for laparoscopic hepatic artery access.

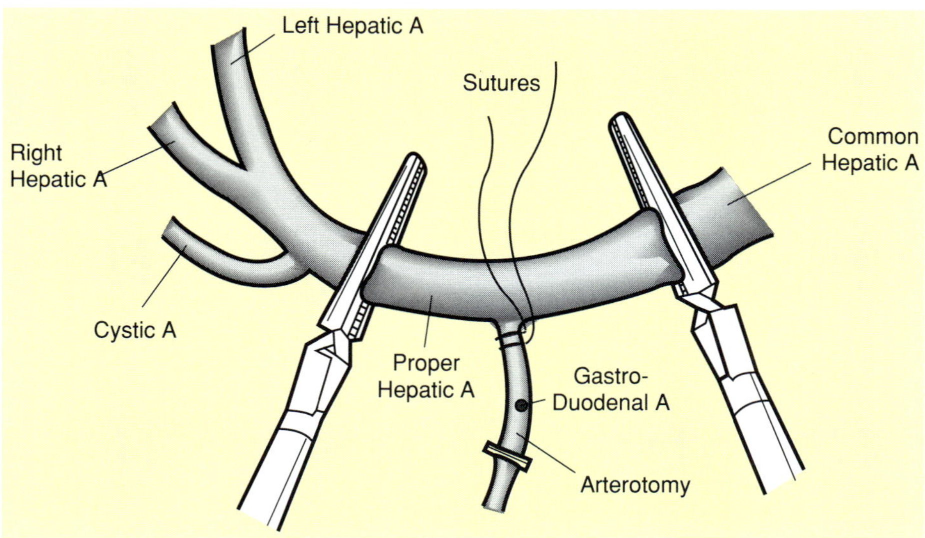

Figure 12.2:   Preparation for catheter introduction.

At this point in the procedure, attention was directed to the placement of the catheter itself. Gentle upward traction was applied to the double-looped silk tie, to expose the gastroduodenal artery. A small transverse arteriotomy was made in the gastroduodenal artery approximately 1 cm distal to its proximal origin. Careful inspection for hemorrhage was carried out to ensure adequate placement of all clamps and clips. A polytetrafluoroethelene catheter was introduced into the abdomen via a cannula site. The catheter tip was directed into the arteriotomy and gingerly advanced towards the common hepatic artery as the retraction on double-looped silk tie was relaxed to ease its passage. The catheter was directed distally into the proper hepatic artery. Once the catheter was in a satisfactory position, the silk tie was tied intracorporeally, and an additional silk tie was passed at the gastroduodenal artery as a second support. The catheter had one additional tie sewn intracorporeally to duodenal serosa as an anchoring stitch. The free end of the catheter was brought out via a cannula site for testing. The laparoscopic bulldog clamps (Birtcher/Solos, Culver City, California, USA) were removed and inspection for bleeding was carried out (Figure 2). Methylene blue was injected into the proximal catheter and the liver was observed to turn appropriately blue in both lobes. The cannula from which the catheter came out of the abdomen was carefully removed, leaving the catheter intact, and a subcutaneous pocket was fashioned at this site. The reservoir was fitted to the catheter end, and the device was placed and sutured inside the subcutaneous pocket. A standard laparoscopic cholecystectomy was then performed with an intraoperative cholangiogram, to avoid the risk of post-hepatic artery chemotherapy-induced cholecystitis. Having checked the abdominal cavity fully for bleeding, the cannulas were removed under direct vision. All fascia were reapproximated at the 10 mm sites and the skin was closed subcuticularly. Our patient was extubated in the operating room and transferred to the intensive care unit in a stable satisfactory condition. Hepatic artery regional chemotherapy infusion with 5 FU was commenced 15 minutes after surgery.

Postoperatively, our first patient initially did somewhat poorly secondary to systemic chemotherapy effects (given as an addition to the regional chemotherapy) and poor self-motivation. The patient was eventually discharged home on the 23rd postoperative day, after which a nurse continued to check on him daily at home. Six months after surgery, computed tomography scan of the patient's abdomen shows no evidence of liver metastasis, and his blood tests confirm normal liver function. He is currently undergoing external pelvic radiation treatment for the primary tumor. Even though the prognosis is still poor, we feel that the patient has been undergoing effective palliative treatment.

Other cases

The procedure has now been performed on five more patients. Three had metastatic colon carcinoma, one had diffuse hepatoma, while the other had metastatic breast cancer and is now our first choice for non-resectable liver carcinoma.

The treatment of hepatic malignancy, whether primary or metastatic, is difficult to manage. There is evidence that regional chemotherapy may help the regression of tumor mass. Klopp and colleagues were the first to propose regional chemotherapy in the treatment of any type of isolated malignancy in 1950[6], and the concept was first applied to hepatic malignancy in 1963[7]. Other anecdotal reports followed, but 1970 saw the publication of a landmark work by Watkins and colleagues[1]. They described significant tumor regression with the permanent hepatic arterial infusion device, and also gave the first detailed description of the open operative technique still used today. Overall, the most important result was the realization that higher doses of chemotherapeutic drug levels could successfully be delivered to the liver with fewer systemic side-effects. However, the placement of these permanent infusion devices requires a formal laparotomy, with its additional morbidity to the patient.

In 1970, Massey and colleagues reported a percutaneous, interventional radiological technique to achieve regional hepatic chemotherapy in a less invasive way[2]. Unfortunately this method is associated with all the complications inherent in arterial cannulization in an extremity, and access is usually for limited infusion periods only, requiring removal of the catheter and reinsertion if any additional dosing or therapy is needed.

Conclusion

The challenge for the oncologist is to obtain long-term access to the hepatic arterial system with the least insult to the patient. The laparoscopic approach may provide the solution. Currently our experience is somewhat limited because of the paucity of suitable patients for this form of therapy. Our patient was the first person subjected to this approach, and all we can currently do is to report the results, but with more investigation laparoscopy may provide a more subtle approach for regional hepatic chemotherapy.

References

1   Watkins E, Khazei AM and Nahra KS (1970) Surgical basis for arterial infusion chemotherapy of disseminated carcinoma of the liver. *Surg Gyn Onc.* **130**: 581–605.

2   Massey WH *et al.* (1971) Hepatic artery infusion for metastatic malignancy using percutaneously placed catheters. *Am J Surg*, **121**: 160–4.

3   Chang AE, Schnieder PD and Sugarbaker PH (1987) A prospective randomized trial of regional vs systemic continuous 5-FU chemotherapy in the treatment of colorectal metastasis. *Ann Surg.* **206**: 685–93.

4   Wageman LD, Kemeny MM and Leong L (1990) A prospective, randomized evaluation of the treatment of colorectal cancer metastatis to the liver. *J Clin Oncol.* **8**: 1885–93.

5   Martin JK, O'Connell MJ and Weiland HS (1990) Intra-arterial floxuridine vs systemic flurouracil for hepatic metastases from colorectal cancer. *Arch Surg.* **125**: 1022–7.

6   Klopp CT *et al.* (1950) Fractionated intra-arterial cancer, chemotherapy with methyl bis amine hydrochloride; a preliminary report. *Ann Surg.* **132**: 811–32.

7   Sullivan RD *et al.* (1963) Continuous arterial infusion chemotherapy of human liver cancer using 5-fluro-2'deoxyuridine: autodetoxification studies and clinical effects. *Proc Am Ass Cancer Res.* **4**: 66.

13

Port-site metastasis

RAGHU S SAVALGI and R DAVID ROSIN

Introduction

In 1870 Reincke[1] reported two cases in which tumors developed at the sites of paracentesis for ascites due to peritoneal carcinomatosis. History was repeated in a different context when two cases of port-site metastasis were reported in 1933[2]. In the last 200 years tumor spread has remained a difficult phenomenon to understand, and minimal access surgery has added several more questions.

Port-site metastasis has gained the attention not only of surgeons performing minimal access surgery, but also of the media. Performing an operation for a benign condition is quite different from performing one for a malignant condition. Patients suffering from malignant conditions may not value the advantages of minimal access surgery if there is an increased risk of tumor spread and less likelihood of cure.

The phenomenon of port-site metastasis should be studied in conjunction with tumor biology. Here, therefore, we give a brief review of the principles of tumor spread, followed by an account of three cases of port-site metastasis and two cases of cutaneous metastasis following conventional surgery for comparison. Some of these cases had previously been operated on by other surgeons, but were seen and operated by us during their follow-up.

General aspects of tumor spread

Metastasis is defined as the transfer of disease from one organ or part thereof to another not directly connected with it[3]. This is due to the transfer of malignant cells, which is one of the main problems in oncological surgery. There are five main steps involved in the tumor spread:

1   infiltration of surrounding tissue and penetration of lymphatics and blood vessels
2   release of malignant cells (singly or in groups) to the circulation
3   survival of malignant cells in the circulation
4   arrest of malignant cells in the capillary beds of distant organs
5   penetration of vasculature and or lymphatics followed by growth of malignant cells.

The pathogenesis of tumor invasion is not very well understood. It may occur as a result of:

- mechanical pressure

- release of lytic enzymes

- increased motility of malignant cells. Cinematography has shown that tumor cells are capable of active movement and migration. Autocrine motility factor can stimulate the motility of cells.

Transcelomic spread is well recognized[4]. When a tumor invades the serosal layer of a viscus, it excites an inflammatory response which leads to effusion. Malignant cells can become entangled with the fibrinous exudate; they can also become detached and be swept away into the peritoneal cavity by serous fluid. They settle widely on its wall, proliferate and give rise to innumerable seedlings. The commonest examples of transcelomic spread is seen in the peritoneal cavity in cases of primary gastric, colonic and ovarian carcinomata. The greater omentum can become heavily infiltrated. Metastases are common in the pouch of Douglas due to a gravitational effect. Transpleural spread occurs in some cases of lung and breast cancer.

Metastasis by implantation on epithelial surfaces

Another method of spread is the inoculation metastasis by implantation of detached tumor cells on epithelial surfaces[5]. There are reported cases of carcinoma spreading from one lip to the other, from one vocal cord to the other, or from one side of the vulva to the other. Secondary growths in the hollow epithelial viscera at a distance from the primary growth have been attributed to surface implantation of tumor fragments transported within cavities of viscera, eg from one lung to the other, from one part of the alimentary tract to another intraluminally, from the gall bladder to the intestine, from ovary to uterus via the tube, and from the renal pelvis and ureter to the bladder.

Inoculation metastasis can occur but it is not common as there are several physiological factors which prevent it. The presence of a rich bacterial flora on the skin, the diminished viability of fragments of tumor and the absence of breaches in healthy epithelial surfaces make inoculation metastasis uncommon. Before concluding that a metastasis results purely from inoculation, it is very important to exclude multiple primary growths and metastases by other routes (transcelomic, lymphatic and blood-borne). Multifocal tumor formation is responsible for most cases of contact cancer.

Dormant tumors

Metastases may appear several years after a primary tumor has been resected. This feature of dormancy is most often seen in carcinoma of the breast and malignant melanoma[4]. The patient may develop metastases 35 years after excision of the primary tumor. The patient usually remains well during the dormant period. There may be no local recurrence. The appearance of metastases may have no precipitating factor. However, it may follow a severe illness, an operation or psychological stress. The disease may progress rapidly once the metastases have appeared. The natural history of most cancers in relation to tumor spread is still poorly understood.

Surgical transplantation and inoculation of tumors

The intentional transplantation of tumors in human beings would constitute a serious criminal offence. In the 19th century, however, such experiments were conducted by some surgeons, who transplanted skin tumor nodules into normal skin[5]. One case was reported where a tumor from one breast was transplanted into the normal breast. These experiments show that it is feasible surgically to transplant tumors into a normal area.

Metastases caused by surgical inoculation at incision sites have been reported over many years. Mayo[6] reported recurrent tumors at suture sites following gastrectomy for carcinoma of the stomach. Kettle[7] reported a metastasis at the puncture site of needle aspiration of a suspected liver abscess. German[8] viewed metastasis from endometrial tumors at the operation site as secondary to the implantation of cells. However, Nicholson[9] believed it to be due to metaplastic change in celomic tissue.

There has been considerable controversy about the presence of malignant cells in the peritoneum following operations for oncological conditions. Moore and colleagues[10] reported that the peritoneal lavage fluid following operations for malignant conditions of the stomach, colon, rectum, ovary, uterus and cervix contained malignant cells. If the colorectal tumors were inoperable, 95% of the cases contained malignant cells, in comparison with 17.5% of operable cases. Juhl and colleagues[11] used immuno-cytochemical techniques and showed that 39% of patients operated for carcinoma of the stomach, colon, rectum and pancreas had intraperitoneal malignant cells. They also showed a direct correlation between the stage of cancer and the presence of intraperitoneal malignant cells. It is not clear whether these cells play a role in implantation metastasis, as wound recurrence is not as high as these quoted figures.

There has been much debate about the viability of disseminated neoplastic cells especially in the lumen of the large intestine. Rosenberg and coworkers[12] doubted that this could be the case for exfoliated cells found in the lumen of the bowel in the case of colorectal cancer. However, Umpelby and colleagues[13] reported that exfoliated cells in the intestinal lumen recovered in the same conditions had an overall viability rate of 90% irrespective of the size of the tumor, Dukes' staging or histological grading. They also showed that cells can grow in a culture medium for as long as 10 days and, if injected into the tail vein of immunodepressed mice, can cause pulmonary tumors. Tanida and colleagues[14] showed that neoplastic cells disseminated in the peritoneum from gastric cancers can remain viable. This has been reconfirmed by Iitsuka and coworkers[15], using the technique of H^3 thymidine incorporation.

Case reports

The following five cases of metastasis following surgery illustrate port-site problems.

Case 1

A 52-year-old woman was extensively investigated by gastroenterology physicians and gynecologists for abdominal pain over a period of more than two years. The only positive finding was the presence of gall stones, and some of her symptoms were attributable to these. She underwent an elective laparoscopic cholecystectomy using the four-port technique. During laparoscopy no associated pathology was discovered. A Redivac drain was inserted in the right lateral port and removed 24 hours after the operation. After being sent home the following day, her symptoms improved. She was reviewed six weeks after the operation and was discharged from the clinic. Twelve months after the operation she presented with pain at the right midclavicular port site. On examination a stitch granuloma was suspected. It was excised and sent for histological examination. This showed adenocarcinoma with a stitch in it, without conclusively suggesting the primary. She underwent further extensive investigations to establish the primary. Computed tomography (CT) scanning of her abdomen suggested an ovarian primary. We performed a diagnostic laparoscopy which confirmed advanced ovarian tumor with extensive intra-abdominal metastases.

Case 2

A 72-year-old man presented with hematemesis. Endoscopy revealed ulceration on the posterior wall of the stomach. The biopsies showed stromal cell tumor of the stomach. He underwent laparoscopic partial gastrectomy[16]. The tumor was removed through the port in the left hypochondrium. The retrieval bag burst while removing the tumor. Four months after the operation he presented with a nodule at the infra-umbilical port site. This was excised and sent for histological study which showed a metastatic deposit of stromal cell tumor. The CT scan of his abdomen confirmed extensive intra-abdominal metastases. He later developed a metastasis in the extracted port site as well.

Case 3

A 56-year-old man underwent laparoscopic anterior resection. During his follow-up his serum CEA was found to be rising. Twelve months after the operation he was found to have a recurrence at the anastamotic site and clinically palpable lumps in the abdominal wall. The CT scan and second laparotomy confirmed extensive intra-abdominal metastases in addition to metastases in the abdominal wall.

Case 4

A 71-year-old woman underwent conventional anterior resection for carcinoma of the rectum. Eight years later she was found to have a recurrence at the site of anastamosis and underwent another resection by conventional technique. Hemorrhage occurred during the second operation and a drain was inserted. Two years later she presented with a metastastic nodule between the main incision scar and the drain site in the left iliac fossa. This was excised under general anesthetic.

Case 5

An 88-year-old man presented with peritonitis. A CT scan revealed a collection in left paracolic gutter, the aspiration of which showed pus. He underwent conventional left hemicolectomy and resection of the adherent small bowel for a perforated Dukes' C1 adenocarcinoma of the colon. Six months after the initial operation he presented with a metastasis at the aspiration site, which was excised. Nine months after the operation he presented with a metastatic deposit at the site of main incision which was also excised. Despite all these recurrences the patient clinically remained well for his age and condition when he was seen nine months after the operation.

Port-site metastasis

Port-site metastasis may be the most obvious but not the only problem: patients may also have extensive metastases within the abdomen. We have used the term 'port-site metastasis' in the past[2]. In this chapter and our previous work on this subject, 'metastases following minimal access surgery' is probably a better term and allows a broader view of the subject. However, there is a need for more extensive research in this area as a number of questions pertaining to the mechanism of these recurrences, still need to be answered.

The simplest explanation of the problem is that malignant cells could be transferred to the port site during the operation and give rise to port-site metastases. However, the real problem may be more complex. In case 1, the patient had a Redivac drain in the right lateral port for 24 hours but developed the port-site metastasis in the midclavicular port site. In case 2, the tumor was removed through the left lateral port site, but the metastasis was seen initially in the umbilical port site which was used only for passing the telescope. In case 3, one of the metastases in the abdominal wall was away from the port site. The site of metastasis in relation to the use of the port appears to be unpredictable in these cases. There is a need for studies to evaluate whether there is any relationship between a particular use of a port and metastasis.

In cases 1 to 3, it is difficult to conclude that the port-site metastasis was purely an inoculation metastasis introduced via the port as the patients had extensive metastases in the abdomen. The transcelomic and lymphatic routes cannot be excluded. It remains to be seen how many of such cases reported in the future will be purely inoculation metastasis at the port site or part of a widespread disease. In case 1, the histology of the gall bladder was normal. Others have reported port-site metastasis after removing gall bladders with histological evidence of adenocarcinoma[17]. It is not clear whether port-site metastasis is dependent on the quantity of tumor cells implanted at the port site. It may be dependent on both 'seed and soil'.

It is conceivable that difficulties in surgical dissection and tumor removal may play a role in cutaneous metastasis. However, in case 1 no dissection was performed near the then-unknown tumor in the ovaries. In case 2, the tumor was removed through the left lateral port although the metastasis was initially seen near the umbilicus. In case 3, there was a metastasis some distance from the port site. Therefore one cannot presume that difficulties in dissection and the tumor removal are the sole contributors to port-site metastasis. The effect of an increased intra-abdominal pressure on malignant cell dispersion in the abdomen, cell motility and cell permeation are still unknown.

The interval between the original operation and the discovery of cutaneous metastasis is variable: in cases 1 and 3 it was 12 months; in case 2 it was four months; in case 4 it was eight years after the first operation and four years after the second operation: and in case 5 it was six months for the first metastasis, nine months for the second. Cava and colleagues[18] reported a subcutaneous metastasis seven days after laparoscopy in a patient with adenocarcinoma of the stomach. Malignant cells can remain dormant in patients presenting with metastasis after a considerable interval. This warrants long-term follow-up of patients to establish what percentage of patients develop port-site metastases.

Drains are known to predispose to metastases. The peritoneal fluid containing malignant cells may provide a bigger dose of inoculation for a longer time at the drain site. It is not clear whether malignant cells survive longer in wounds of smaller diameter which would be relevant to port sites. It is also not clear whether the smooth surface of the ports has any effect on cell survival. Preventive factors such as washing the port site with locally acting chemotherapeutic agents need to be evaluated.

Conclusion

For many years it has been recognized that local factors are important in determining the sites of metastasis[19]. Murthy and colleagues[20] showed experimentally that the frequency of tumor implantation is greater when cancer cells are presented to wounds in their early rather than late stages of healing. Tumor cells reaching the operative sites bind to fibrin and become entrapped in the fibrin gel. These newly implanted cells may benefit from the surgically induced depression of host immunity and the release of growth factors from the regenerating tissues. These factors may play a role in the formation of port-site metastasis. It is more worrying if minimal access surgery leads to widespread metastasis for whatever reason and port-site metastasis may be only the most visible (rather than the most serious) problem. It is not yet known whether the frequency of metastasis is higher after minimal access surgery than conventional surgery. Randomized clinical studies are still awaited. We hope that clinicians and basic scientists will contribute to the understanding of 'metastases following minimal access surgery' which are detrimental to the practice and survival of laparoscopic oncological surgery.

References

1   Reincke J (1870) Metastasis following paracentesis. *Virchows Arch*. **51**: 391.

2   Savalgi RS and Rosin RD (1993) Evaluation of port site metastasis following laparoscopic operations. *Min Inv Ther*. **2** (Suppl. 1): 34.

3   Hart IR (1991) The spread of tumours. In: Franks LM and Teich NM (eds.) *Introduction to the Cellular and Molecular Biology of Cancer*, 2nd edn. Oxford University Press, Oxford. pp. 31–48.

4   Walter JB and Israel MS (1979). *General Pathology*. Churchill Livingstone, Edinburgh. pp. 3259–66.

5   Willis RA (1973) *The Spread of Tumours in the Human Body*, 3rd edn. London, Butterworths. pp. 61–70.

6   Mayo WJ (1913) Recurrence of tumour at suture line. *JAMA*. **60**: 512–13.

7   Kettle EH (1912) *The Pathology of Tumours*. Lewis, London. p. 25.

8   German WJ (1928) Endometrial tumours at the operations scars. *Surg Obstet Gyn*. **47**: 710–13.

9   Nicholson GW (1926) A review on the metastasis of endometrial tumours. *J Obstet Gyn Br Emp*. **33**: 620–4.

10   Moore GE *et al*. (1961). Assessment of the exfoliation of tumour cells into the body cavities. *Surg Gyn Obstet*. **112**: 469.

11 Juhl H, Stritzel M. Wroblewski A *et al.* (1994) Immunocytochemical detection of micro-metastatic cells: comparative evaluation of findings in the peritoneal and pancreatic cancer patients. *Int J Cancer.* **57**: 330–5.

12 Rosenberg IL, Russell CW and Giles GR (1978) Cell viability studies on the exfoliated colonic cancer cell. *Br J Surg.* **65**: 188–90.

13 Umpleby HC, Fermor B, Symes MO *et al.* (1984) Viability of exfoliated colorectal carcinoma cells. *Br J Surg.* **71**: 659–63.

14 Tanida O, Kancshima S, Iisuka Y *et al.* (1982) Viability of intraperitoneal free cancer cells in patients with gastric cancer. *Acta Cytol.* **26**: 681–7.

15 Iisuka Y, Kaneshima S, Tanida O *et al.* (1979) Intra-peritoneal cancer cells and their viability in gastric cancer. *Cancer.* **44**: 1476–80.

16 Savalgi RS and Rosin RD (1993) Laparoscopic partial gastrectomy for leiomyoma of the stomach. *Surg Endosc.* 7 257.

17 Nduka CC, Monson JRT, Menzies-Gow N *et al.* (1994) Abdominal wall metastases following laparoscopy. *Br J Surg.* **81**: 648–52.

18 Cava A, Roman J, Gonzalez Quintola A *et al.* (1990) Subcutaneous metastasis following laparoscopy in gastric adenocarcinoma. *Eur J Surg Oncol.* **16**: 373–5.

19 Poste G and Fidler IJ (1982) The pathogenesis of cancer metastasis. *Nature.* **283**: 139–46.

20 Murthy SM, Goldschmidt RA, Rao LN *et al.* (1989) The influence of surgical trauma on experimental metastasis. *Cancer.* **64**: 2035–44.

14

Oncological risks in laparoscopic surgery

JEAN MOUIEL, FRANCESCO CRAFA, RAFFAELE CURSIO,
ROBERT STUBINSKI and JEAN GUGENHEIM

Introduction

The risk of tumor spread by laparoscopy has received increasing attention since the first reports of port-site metastasis after laparoscopic cholecystectomy for unsuspected gall-bladder cancer. Evidence of tumor spread during laparoscopic surgery for cancers of the digestive tract or other organ systems has raised a crucial question:

> Is this phenomenon a consequence of mechanical implantation of cancer cells during laparoscopy as was demonstrated at the very outset of conventional surgery and thus necessitating measures to prevent tumor seeding during laparoscopy, or is there another phenomenon, biologic in nature, for which laparoscopy may be responsible, at least partially, causing a mutation of the neoplastic cells and thus resulting in an increase of the risk of tumor spread?

This chapter addresses the question by comparing data from laparoscopic and conventional procedures. A summary of the ways in which tumors may spread is followed by a discussion of how such dissemination may be prevented.

Review of cases

In order to emphasize the risk of port-site metastasis and tumor spread during laparoscopic oncological surgery, we have reviewed the clinical reports published in the international literature between 1991 and 1994. We have also included ten additional patients who have come to our attention in a confidential manner through personal communications.

Laparoscopic cholecystectomy[1–14]

In all cases, neoplasms were unsuspected before laparoscopic surgery. Sixteen of the 17 reported cases were women, and the mean age was 55 ± 2 years (mean $\pm$ SEM., range 40–70 years). In eight of the 17 referred cases there was a wide variety of difficulties during the operation, including difficult extraction with associated biliary and stone spillage from the gall bladder, rupture of the gall bladder and abdominal wall contamination. Postoperative specimen examination revealed a T1 carcinoma in two cases, T2 carcinoma in one case and T3 carcinoma in 14 cases. The carcinoma was poorly differentiated in two cases and moderately differentiated in three. The mean time for clinical tumor relapse was 81 ± 13 days (mean $\pm$ sem., range 21–240 days). An early recurrence (21–65 days) was observed in nine cases; in five cases recurrence occurred between 65 and 109 days, and the remaining patients had a recurrence between days 109 and 241. In six patients the tumor recurrence was manifested as a single nodule; in five patients, two metastases were described; and in the remaining patients there was a diffuse spread of the disease. The mean diameter of the recurrence was 2 ± 0.7 cm (mean $\pm$ sem). Port sites were involved in 10 patients: there was port-site and associated peritoneal dissemination in one patient, port-site and peritoneal involvement in three cases, and port-site hepatic and peritoneal dissemination in one. Subsequently three patients underwent radiotherapy, six had chemotherapy, and one patient had the tumor excised. Death was documented in nine patients, with a mean survival time of 226 ± 41 days (mean $\pm$ sem., range 90–450 days) needs. Berthou and colleagues have also told us of three additional cases of gall-bladder tumor recurrence after laparoscopic cholecystectomy, all following unsuspected T3 tumors[15].

Laparoscopic colorectal surgery[9,13,14,16–18]

Seven reports have come to our attention concerning the recurrence of colorectal cancer after laparoscopic surgery. There were five women and two men, with a mean age of 73 ± 2.8 years (mean $\pm$ sem., range 65–72 years). The tumor site was the rectum in two patients, the right colon in three, and the cecum in two. The histological stage was Dukes' B in one case and Dukes' C in six. Histological analysis of the tumor showed a moderately differentiated tumor in two of the patients. Two Miles resections and five laparoscopically assisted right hemicolectomies were performed. The mean time for tumor recurrence after bowel resection was 124 ± 40 days (mean $\pm$ sem., range 45–300 days). In three patients there was a solitary secondary recurrence, in two cases there were two metastases, in one patient three metastases and in one patient there was a port-site metastasis associated with diffuse tumor spread. The sites of metastases were the port site only in four cases, the mini-laparotomy scar in one patient, and the port site and the perineal scar in one patient; in the remaining patient the port-site localization was associated with hepatic metastases. The reported treatment for these recurrences was radiotherapy in one patient, chemotherapy in another and resection combined with chemotherapy in a third. Two deaths were reported (184 and 270 days, respectively, after the laparoscopic procedures) and one patient is still alive with the disease. Our personal enquiries have yielded data on seven additional cases of colonic tumor recurrence following laparoscopic bowel surgery for Dukes' A, C and D colon cancer[19].

Other carcinomas

Port-site metastases have been observed as a consequence of laparoscopic biopsy for hepatocellular carcinomas[20], after diagnostic laparoscopy for ascites originating from a neoplastic gastric disease[21], after laparoscopic cholecystectomy for a misdiagnosed pancreatic carcinoma[22], after laparoscopic partial gastrectomy for a gastric carcinoma[23], after laparoscopic appendectomy for an unsuspected carcinoma of the appendix[24] and after laparoscopic resection of an ovary for an unsuspected ovarian cancer[25] or for early malignant ovarian tumors[26].

Characteristics of port-site metastasis

The characteristics of port-site metastasis depend on whether the metastasis is associated with other neoplastic disease. The gross appearance of a metastatic nodule without evidence of other recurrence is that of a hard mass, deeply encased in the skin which is taut above it, without concomitant signs of infiltration or inflammation. The average size is between 3 and 4 cm (range 1–8 cm), and the nodules may be single or multiple. The metastasis is located at the site where the trocar was inserted, both if it was inserted perpendicular to the plane of the abdominal wall or if the bayonet technique for trocar insertion was used, or in the mini-laparotomy scar. The parietal peritoneum is perfectly healed and held back by the nodular lesion and would not seem to be the starting point for parietal metastasis. The nodule is therefore strictly intraparietal, consisting of malignant cells enclosed in striated fibromuscular tissue. Having considered the aspects of a single metastasis we have to keep in mind that it is possible to be faced with such a nodule or nodules which are part of a local recurrence, either starting out from the primary tumor and invading the trocar/mini-laparotomy site, or being part of a diffuse recurrence in the setting of massive peritoneal carcinomatosis. It seems possible to distinguish between:

- the single parietal nodule which rapidly appears in less than two months

- the parietal nodules associated with peritoneal carcinomatosis

- metastatic tumor cells appearing later, ie after four months[13].

Observations in open surgery

The development of parietal metastases at the sites of fine needle biopsies, paracentesis, postoperative surgical drains or operation scars was noted a long time ago. There are reports of parietal metastases originating from hepatic[27] and pancreatic[28] neoplasms after diagnostic paracentesis (evaluation of cell characteristics found in ascites aspirates), after fine needle biopsy of a hepatocellular carcinoma[29], and even after transparietal hepatic positioning of a stent under radiological guidance[30]. The mechanism of tumor cell implantation is probably the same for diagnostic paracentesis of malignant ascites as following the positioning of surgical drains in a patient with abdominal malignancy. The appearance of parietal metastases in scars following laparotomy for surgical excision of an abdominal neoplasm was first reported over 80 years ago by Mayo[31], who described the case of one of his patients who underwent gastrectomy for a gastric cancer. Earlier von Mickulicz[32] had described parietal metastasis after exteriorization of a tumoral colonic loop. This operation initially gained popularity because of the low postoperative mortality rate, but was quickly abandoned because of the risk of neoplastic contamination of the surgical scar. More recently, parietal metastases have been reported as taking place after resective surgery for abdominal, digestive, retroperitoneal and gynecological tumors[33–36]. We can therefore conclude that although the development of parietal metastasis has been known for a long time, it is usually neglected in the context of peritoneal carcinomatosis, and in practice only attracts attention if it appears on its own in a patient who has been operated on for curative reasons.

The metastatic potential of malignant tumors

The metastatic potential of malignant tumors is the result of cell dissemination, which depends on the freeing of cancer cells in the original tumor as the result of the break-up of the intercellular bridge framework. Neoplastic cell dissemination specifically with gastrointestinal cancer has been the object of many scientific reports. Particularly with colorectal cancers it has been demonstrated that cancer may disseminate by means of:

- cancer cells circulating in the blood stream and/or the lymphatic vessels

- exfoliated cells in the intestinal lumen

- free cancer cells in the peritoneum.

Cancer cells in the blood stream

Cytological methods after centrifugation may reveal circulating cancer cells in the blood stream[37,38]. High proportions (25–67%) have been demonstrated in the veins draining malignant tumors; in the surrounding veins the proportion is between 5 and 36%. Many reports have suggested that a relationship exists between neoplastic circulating cells and tumor mobilization, tumor stage and grading, and it seems likely that neoplastic cells are continuously freed into the blood steam[39]. However, Engell[40] found no prognostic relationship between such cell dissemination and patient survival, in a series of patients operated on for colorectal cancer and followed up for between five and nine years. Such contradictory facts mean that we must be cautious when interpreting tumor malignancy using cytological methods as a basis, because these techniques can give rise to confusion particularly for hematopoietic cells[39]. This has been proved by the work done by Leather and colleagues of the Phillips group[41] whose immunocytochemical methods confirmed that neoplastic cells do circulate in the tumor drainage veins and in the peripheral blood stream, but who found only 10% of circulating cells instead of the expected 30% despite two of their patients having Dukes' B tumors. These authors also stressed that both vascular and lymphatic dissemination is an intermittent phenomenon and that its frequency is in keeping with the efforts made to find it.

Exfoliated cells in the intestinal lumen

The presence of exfoliated cells in the intestinal lumen has been established for a long time, since free-moving cancerous cells have been found on either side of a tumor in the intestinal lumen and also in the stools[39]. Umpleby and coworkers[42], using vital staining and fluorescein via in vivo washing and ex vivo irrigation of the extremities of the resected bowel, found neoplastic cells in the proximal part of large bowel in 57% of cases, at an average distance of 10.8 cm (range 4–35 cm) from the primary tumor, and in the distal part of the large bowel in 84% of the patients, at an average distance of 7.5 cm (range 3–20 cm) from the neoplasm.

Free cancer cells in the peritoneum

The presence of free cancer cells in the peritoneum was demonstrated by Pomeranz and Garlock[43] who described two cases of invasive cancers; it was also confirmed by Quan[44] who analysed the peritoneal fluid of 133 patients, which proved positive in 15 cases. These facts, which were initially proven for colorectal cancers, were confirmed by Moore and colleagues[45] for the majority of abdominal–perineal malignancies including the stomach, colon, rectum, ovaries, uterus and cervix, when they compared 727 patients operated upon for abdominal–perineal cancer with 166 patients operated upon for benign disease. The analysis of the peritoneal lavage liquid showed that in 95% of cases of inoperable colorectal cancers there were 40% with malignant cells present, whereas in 166 patients operated for resectable colorectal cancers there were only 17.5% with malignant cells. The importance of cellular dissemination of this kind gave rise to further doubts as to the very nature of the cells diagnosed in the earlier studies which used purely cytological methods. However a recent study conducted by Juhl and coworkers[46], who used immunocytological methods, showed the presence of neoplastic cells in the peritoneum of patients with abdominal malignancies (27% for colorectal cancers, 43% for gastric cancers and 58% for pancreatic cancers), with an overall average value of 39%—significantly higher than the amounts detected by conventional cytology. Furthermore, the same authors have established a correlation between the proportion of malignant cells and tumor stage, from 20% for stage I through to 65% for stage IV, depending on the type of the cancer. They have also shown that in the patients in question there were micro-metastases in the bone marrow in almost identical proportions[46–48].

Viability of neoplastic cells

Rosenberg and colleagues[49] doubted the viability of exfoliated neoplastic cells found in the lumen of the bowel in the case of colorectal cancer after studying preoperative intestinal lavage or after washing the operative specimen and using colorimetric methods after preparation, incubation and centrifugation. Umpleby and colleagues, on the other hand, by modifying the technique of centrifugation and using vital color dyes and fluorescein, proved that exfoliated cells in the intestinal lumen, recovered in the same conditions, had an overall viability rate of 90% irrespective of tumor volume, Dukes' stage or histological grading[42]. The same group of authors[50] have shown elsewhere that cells can grow in a culture medium for as long as 10 days and are even able to cause pulmonary tumors when injected into the tail vein of immunosupressed mice. These results have been confirmed by Skipper and colleagues[51]. As regards gastric cancers, the viability of neoplastic cells disseminated in the peritoneum, using colorimetric processes[52], has also been clearly established by Iitsuka and coworkers[53] using the technique of H^3-thymidine incorporation which registered positive in the great majority of cases. Indirect proof of the viability of such cells is offered by immunocytological studies showing the correlation between them and the tumor stage and thus emphasizes their prognostic significance[46].

Tumor development

The frequency of micro-metastases, even in the early stages of the neoplasm, suggests that tumor development occurs in three steps:

1   the closed tumor
2   the open tumor from which hidden micro-metastases originate
3   the tumor with proven metastasis.

The first phase concerns cancers in their initial form; the tumors are usually less than 2 cm in size and can be cured by simple excision. At present little is known about the second phase of hidden micro-metastatic tumors because of the lack of any suitable detecting instruments and also because such dissemination is intermittent and therefore difficult to prove[41]. The hidden phase of micro-metastasis may vary considerably in time, ranging between five and 20 years, and this has generated the idea of dormant tumor cells[54]. This has indeed been proven experimentally and such tumor cell dormancy suggests that after radical treatment of the primary cancer, a metastasis which was unsuspected at the time of the operation may develop several years later. During this interval of time these micro-metastases remain quiescent in a kind of symbiosis with the host organism. It has been suggested that the analysis of the tumor cell cycle can in part explain this phenomenon: in fact there are non-cycling cells in GO–GZ (phase fractions) in most parts of neoplasms which increase in number along with an increase in the tumor size. It has been demonstrated that many tumors are made up of non-cycling cells[54]. Proliferation and dissemination by 'resting' cells is stimulated by immunosuppression, the masking of tumor antigens and mechanical, chemical or surgical trauma as proved experimentally by Fisher and coworkers[55]. In the third phase, the tumor 'opens out', colonizing other parts of the organism. This happens either spontaneously or after the failure of whatever treatment has been applied.

Digestive cancer spread

There are at least five ways in which cancers of the digestive system may spread: directly, lymphatically, hemotologically, intraluminally and intraperitoneally[39]. All have been meticulously studied, especially in the context of colorectal cancer which shall serve as an example. Direct dissemination is influenced by the eccentric radial and longitudinal growth of the tumor which gradually invades all the layers of the intestine and finally invades neighboring organs, some of which are a considerable distance away. Growth is slow, as it may be about two years before the tumor becomes circumferential. This is of practical interest when the serosa is involved as the result of an increased inflammatory reaction with greater cellular exfoliation. The theory of lymphatic spread is the basis of all oncological surgery. In fact lymph-node invasion is progressive, beginning from the paracolic nodes and spreading to the central nodes. Such metastatic tumor cells are common since they have been found (depending on the stage) in 38–60% of cases of colon cancer and in 50–60% of cases of rectal cancer[39], although studies using monoclonal antibodies[56] suggest that this may be an underestimate. Blood-stream dissemination has already been described in the context of cell circulation. Venous invasion as seen in the pathology specimen is particularly common, taking place in some 52% of cases, and is proportional to tumor extension, from 20% of Dukes' stage A, to 47% in Dukes' stage B and up to 64% in Dukes' stage C[39]. This type of venous dissemination explains the frequency of hepatic metastases, found in 30–50% of patients with advanced cancers of which at least two-thirds are not recognized at the time of surgical resection. In addition to the hepatic filter, other organs such as the lungs, the adrenal glands and the kidneys can be colonized. Of great importance is the presence of micro-metastases in the bone marrow[46] in patients with digestive neoplasms, amounting to 34% overall: 25% in patients with gastric cancer, 29% in those with colorectal cancer and 58% in patients with pancreatic cancer. Intraperitoneal dissemination is revealed at advanced stages of cancers by peritoneal, epiploic and visceral nodules associated with ascites. Intraluminal dissemination is responsible for recurrence along suture lines and in areas where surgery has taken place even if the operation seemed to be curative as in cases of Dukes' A lesions.

The importance of cellular exfoliation stressed earlier would certainly explain why the frequency of such local recurrences varies between 2.6 and 32% depending on whether they are isolated or associated with metastatic tumor cells[57,58].

Metastatic development

The mechanisms by which metastases develop have been compared to a 'decathlon' since the selected tumor cells must undergo a series of tests in order to develop a new tumor center at a distance from the primary neoplasm[59]. The starting point of this 'decathlon' is the escape of metastatic cells after loosening their intercellular bonds under the influence of scatter factors. At this point three mechanisms can be used to explain the metastatic disease:

- vascular associated with angiogenesis

- implantation or inoculation

- biological, cellular and/or immunological processes.

The vascular mechanism

The vascular mechanism is common in epithelial cancers which are disseminated via lymph nodes or the blood stream: The liberated neoplastic cells cross the endothelial lining of the blood vessel and invade the blood stream either individually or in small groups. In this phase during the passage through the arteriovenous shunts, the majority of the neoplastic cells die due to a mechanical shock which is a consequence of high blood pressure. It has been estimated that after an intravenous injection of neoplastic cells 50% die within four hours and 99.5% within 24 hours. This mechanical phenomenon is associated with the action of the immunocompetent cells (NK and T cytotoxic lymphocytes) present in the host, whose task is to destroy neoplastic cells. A few cells survive and these can aggregate with platelets to form neoplastic emboli. Protected in this manner, such cells in contact with the capillary endothelium lodge at this level and multiply by neoangiogenesis in the selected parenchyma[60].

Tumor implantation

The mechanism of tumor implantation was described at the turn of the century by Ryall[61], who reported several examples of metastasis by implantation taking place after digestive or breast cancer operations. In anecdotal articles he described the presence of cancer cells on the scalpel and under the nails of surgeons who did not yet wear gloves. This led to surgeons all over the world changing their instruments after performing a biopsy of a malignant tumor. In the field of conventional surgery there is no lack of proof of tumor cell implantation on an anastomosis: Goligher[39] described this occurring after resection of a colorectal cancer, on the rectal stump after a Hartman operation, on the abdominal wall (for which he reported six patients) and in one case of a patient who had a misdiagnosed cancer who underwent hemorrhoidectomy. This latter localization has been confirmed by Killingback and colleagues[62] who reported five patients with metastases on the scars of hemorrhoidectomies, an anal fistula and an anal fissure. Since then a large number of studies have brought further confirmation of cases of metastases by implantation taking place in open surgery, thus emphasizing the circumstances during operations which are able to cause massive cellular dissemination. Following an anastomotic fistula[63], rates of local recurrence were reported to be as high as 46.9%, compared with 18.5% when no fistula is present. Similarly, rates of between 20 and 51% were noted when the tumor was perforated during surgery as compared with a rate of 11–21% when perforation was not observed[57,64,65]. Mere trauma has been implicated as being responsible for an increased rate of tumor growth, and this has been confirmed experimentally[55].

Biological factors

Biological factors which give rise to metastasis are poorly understood, although much research has been carried out in three main fields:

1   cells, where biological identity has been established between inflammatory reaction and tumor development with growth and antigenic factors[56] being transported by platelets and the secretion of protease-like enzymes by macrophages or tumor cells
2   genetics, where genetic instability causing chromosomal changes and mutations explain heterogeneity of the tumor cells and the selections of those prone to metastasize
3   immunology, where the ability of certain cancer cells to escape the host's control and defence system as represented by NK cells, macrophages and cytotoxic lymphocytes show that we are beginning to have an insight into how a tumor evolves in relation to the host and into the very particular phenomenon of cancer cell dormancy.

Summing up, it appears today that cancer 'sows everywhere' and that metastatic implantation follows. Paget's law[67] concerning 'seed and soil' stressed the importance of environmental factors under the influence of growth and also angiogenic factors. In this fashion the same laws have to be invoked in laparoscopic as in conventional surgery in order to explain metastasis taking place after digestive cancer treatment: local recurrence as the result of implantation of exfoliated cells which has been proven in open surgery[68] corresponds to malignant intraperitoneal cells penetrating cannula sites after laparoscopic surgery. Indeed the friction of the tissue around the trocar/cannula caused by frequent surgical maneuvers is the cause of an inflammatory reaction which is constituted of clots made of fibrin, fibronectin and platelets in its center. Cancer cells disseminated in the peritoneum or originating in intraluminal exfoliation as a result of the manipulation of the tumor are trapped in this gel which offers on the one hand a protective barrier against the host's defence mechanism and on the other nutritional surroundings very suitable for cellular development by producing factors of tumor growth and angiogenesis. Furthermore the implantation of cells circulating in the capillary and subperitoneal lymphatic network is facilitated by the inflammatory reaction of the port sites thus playing the part of a fixation 'abscess' or a trauma[55]. Finally, the process of expansion by neoangiogenesis[66] is responsible for the growth of metastasis.

Mechanisms of possible tumor dissemination in laparoscopy

The creation of a pressurized operative field with carbon dioxide being insufflated and continuously renewed to compensate the action of lavage–aspiration undoubtedly favours the dissemination of free micrometastatic tumor cells in the peritoneal cavity and more specifically at the port sites and at the mini-laparotomy extraction site. Indeed the pneumoperitoneum of 14 mmHg as used in normal laparoscopic procedures favours capillary stasis and as a consequence offers a further factor for facilitating the metastatic implantation of neoplastic cells in the blood stream. Manipulating a poorly isolated tumor, the absence of any ligature around the vessels and the length of the operation further increase the release of neoplastic cells and facilitates their dissemination. It must be added that the tearing of the tissues, the difficulties of obtaining lymphostasis and the use of mechanical suture clips which crush the lympho–venous structures all play an equally important role. Extraction by 'milking' of an organ through a small size mini-laparotomy can also cause parietal contamination as the result of direct contamination aggravated by the exsufflation of the pneumoperitoneum containing cells trapped in a closed atmosphere[14,70]. Is a mechanical action of this kind accompanied by corresponding biological action? In other words, can the pneumoperitoneum give rise to a secretion of factors following growth and neoangiogenesis, immunosuppression, and even genetic amplification or cellular mutation? At the moment there is no reason for thinking so, and the first studies which have appeared suggest, on the contrary, that laparoscopy causes less immunosuppression than conventional surgery[71]. Indeed, published cases of parietal recurrence, even if they only represent the 'tip of the iceberg', are about the same as with those of open surgery. With regard to colorectal cancer, for example, Goligher[39] reported only six cases of parietal contamination in a series of 1640 patients, while Hughes and coworkers[36] cited only 11 cases of 1603 (0.69%). These values may be compared with those from surveys carried out by the American Society of Colo-Rectal Surgeons (ASCRS). Ramos and colleagues[72], from the group of Beart[73], reported a prospective study based on the registry of the ASCRS which began in 1991. The registry contained 252 cases of cancer which were operated on by laparoscopy. Among 208 follow-up reports, three cases of port-site recurrence were observed (1.44%). Two of these three reported cases were associated with diffuse peritoneal carcinomatosis, hence the incidence of port-site recurrence was 0.49%. In all three of these patients the stage was Dukes' C and recurrence occurred at 6, 8, and 21 months postoperatively. Wexner and Cohen[70] performed an enquiry among 635 surgeons of the ASCRS about laparoscopic bowel resection for neoplastic disease: nine cases were reported to have had early local recurrence after curative rectal cancer resection; nine more had early local recurrence after curative resection of colon cancer and five had early port-site recurrence. They concluded laparoscopy does not appear to bring added risk, but the time-span for observing such new operational procedures is at present too short. Without doubt the rate of recurrence is almost certainly influenced by other factors, eg the experience of the surgeon. For open surgery, Phillips and colleagues[57] observed that the tumor recurrence rate was between 5 and 20% for the 20 surgeons taking part in the survey[74].

Preventive measures

Preventive oncological precautions which are habitually taken in conventional surgery[39] must not be forgotten. The no-touch technique[75], with limited manipulation of the tumor, elective ligature of the vessels at their origin, ligature of the colon above and below the tumor and packing of the tumor all represent means of preventing intraperitoneal neoplastic cell dissemination. The preoperative washout and peroperative chemical and mechanical irrigation ensure that exfoliated cells in the intestinal lumen are destroyed. Doubt remains however, about the effectiveness of the three commonly used tumoricidal agents, ie povidone–iodine, sodium hypochlorite and chlorhexidine cetrimide. All three reach 100% tumor cell death in vitro with an exposure time of five minutes, but their efficacy is less in vivo[76]. Research is currently under way in order to evaluate the efficacy of adjuvant chemotherapy either in the peritoneum[77] or in the intestinal lumen and by either the intraportal route or by means of a peripheral vein. As yet the experiments have not been conclusive[58]. In the same way, intraoperative radiotherapy or photodynamic therapy may be effective against cancer cells free in the peritoneum[58]. Specific precautions have to be taken for laparoscopic surgery and must, therefore, be deduced from the rules as set out above[70,72,78–80]. It is easy not to manipulate the tumor traumatically, to ligate the vessels and exclude the tumor. Bagging the tumor at the moment of removal remains a necessity, as is the protection of the abdominal wall during a mini-laparotomy by plastic draping in order to prevent its contamination. At the end of the operation it is advisable to carry out a carbon dioxide aspiration rather than brutal exsufflation as the former may prevent possible viral contamination[81]. Finally the use of chemotherapy, as suggested by Moertel and colleagues[82] for colon cancers, or the use of preoperative radiotherapy as described by the European Organization for Research and Treatment of Cancer[83] for rectal cancers, is a wise precaution. Research, however, needs to be stimulated. Apart from the basic cancer research which can answer some of the questions, surgeons will need to study in a prospective and coordinated multicentric manner three types of procedures in order to avoid neoplastic cell dissemination:

1   abdominal wall lifting devices which abolish the need for a pneumoperitoneum and thus avoid a potential source of mechanical dissemination
2   the use of tumoricidal agents for washing the port sites which must be fully repaired in order to avoid inflammatory reactions
3   intraperitoneal chemotherapy which could be combined with either intraportal or general chemotherapy.

Conclusion

Oncological risks following laparoscopic surgery, as evident from the appearance of port-site metastasis, can be clearly and logically explained in the study of metastatic dissemination as being essentially mechanical in origin. Hidden micro-metastases may cause recurrence which may in turn be followed by laparoscopic procedures which do not respect the normal rules of oncology. Such facts should stimulate research, encourage surgeons to undertake surgery of this kind in recognized centers in accordance with carefully defined multi-center protocols and to apply the rules for conventional surgery to minimal access surgery[84,85]. This is the price to pay if patients are not to be penalized by being treated by an 'immediate' minimal access procedure, which respects the corporeal scheme, reducing the amount of pain, shortening the hospital stay and facilitating the rehabilitation, but with disastrous consequences resulting in the end being 'long-term maximally invasive'.

It would appear with experience that there is no increased risk in minimal access oncological surgery.

References

1   Gornish AL, Averbach D and Schwartz MR (1991) Carcinoma of the gallbladder found during laparoscopic cholecystectomy: a case report and review of the literature. *J Laparoendosc Surg*. **1**: 361–7.

2   Drouard F, Delamarre J and Capron JP (1991) Cutaneous seeding of gallbladder cancer after laparoscopic cholecystectomy. *N Eng J Med*. **325**: 1316.

3   Barsoum GH and Windsor CWO (1992) Parietal seeding of carcinoma of the gallbladder after laparoscopic cholecystectomy. *Br J Surg*. **79**: 846 (Letter).

4   Pezet D *et al*. (1992) Parietal seeding of carcinoma of the gallbladder after laparoscopic cholecystectomy. *Br J Surg*. **79**: 230.

5   Landen SM (1993) Laparoscopic surgery and tumor seeding. *Surg*. **144**: 131–2.

6   Berthet B, Le Treut YP and Assadourian R (1993) Métastase sur le site d'extraction laparoscopique des cancers de la vésicule de diagnostic post-opératoire. *Lyon Chir*. **89**: 50–1.

7   Fong, Y *et al.* (1993) Gallbladder cancer discovered during laparoscopic surgery. *Arch Surg.* **128**: 1054–6.

8   Fligelstone, L *et al.* (1993) Tumor inoculation during laparoscopy. *Lancet.* **342**: 368 (Letter).

9   O'Rourke N *et al.* (1993) Tumor inoculation during laparoscopy. *Lancet.* **342**: 368 (Letter).

10   Clair DG, Lautz DB and Brooks DC (1993) Rapid development of umbilical metastases after laparoscopic cholecystectomy for unsuspected gallbladder carcinoma. *Surg.* **113**: 355–8.

11   Lucciarini P, Konigsrainer A and Eberl T (1993) Tumor inoculation during laparoscopic cholecystectomy. *Lancet.* **342**: 59.

12   Weiss S, Wengert P and Harkavy S (1994) Incisional recurrence of gallbladder cancer after laparoscopic cholecystectomy. *Gastrointest Endosc.* **40**, 2: 244–6.

13   Bouvier S and GRECCO Group (1994) Metastases sur les trajets de trocars après traitement coelio-chirurgical de tumeur digestives. *J Coelio Chir.* **10**: 13–22.

14   Nduka CC, Monson JRT, Menzies-Gow N *et al.* (1994) Abdominal wall metastasis following laparoscopy. *Br J Surg.* **81**: 648–52.

15   Berthou JC, Kestens J and Leroy J. Personal communication.

16   Guillou PJ, Darzi A and Monson JRT (1993) Experience with laparoscopic surgery for malignant disease. *Surg Onc.* **2**: 43–9.

17   Fusco MA and Paluzzi MW (1993) Abdominal wall recurrence after laparoscopic assisted colectomy for adenocarcinoma of the colon. *Dis Colon Rec.* **36**: 858–61.

18   Alexander RJT, Jacques BC and Mitchell KG (1993) Laparoscopically assisted colectomy and wound recurrence (Letter). *Lancet.* 1993; **341**: 249–50.

19   Berthou JC *et al.* Personal communication.

20   Russi EG *et al.* (1992) Unusual relapse of hepatocellular carcinoma. *Cancer.* **15**: 1483–7.

21   Cava A *et al.* (1990) Subcutaneous metastasis following laparoscopy in gastric adeno-carcinoma. *Eur J Surg Oncol.* **16**: 63–7.

22   Siriwardena A and Samarji WN (1993) Cutaneous tumour seeding from a previously undiagnosed pancreatic carcinoma after laparoscopic cholecystectomy. *Ann R Coll Surg Eng.* **75**: 199–200.

23   Savalgi RS and Rosin RD (1993) Laparoscopic partial gastrectomy for leiomyoma of the stomach. *Surg Endosc.* **7** (3): 257.

24   Gould R. Personal communication.

25   Crouet H and Heron JF (1991) Dissémination du cancer de l'ovaire lors de la chirurgie coelioscopique: un danger réel. *Presse Médicale.* **20**: 1738–9.

26   Gleeson NC *et al.* (1993) Abdominal wall metastasis from ovarian cancer after laparoscopy. *Am J Obstet Gyn.* **169**: 522–3.

27   McGrath FP, Gibney RG and Rowley VA (1991) Case report: cutaneous seeding following fine needle biopsy of colonic liver metastases. *Clin Radiol.* 1991; **43**: 130–1.

28   Rashleigh-Belcher HJC, Russel RCG and Lees WR (1986) Cutaneous seeding of pancreatic carcinoma by fine needle aspiration biopsy. *Br J Radiol.* **59**: 182–3.

29   Quaghebeur G *et al.* (1991) Implantation of hepatocellular carcinoma after percutaneous needle biopsy. *J R Coll Surg Edin.* **36**: 127.

30   Olega JA *et al.* (1980) Extension of neoplasm along the tract of a transhepatic tube. *Am J Radiol.* **135**: 841–2.

31   Mayo WJ (1913) Recurrence of tumour at suture line. *JAMA.* **60**: 512–13.

32   von Mikulicz J (1903) Small contributions to the surgery of the intestinal tract. *Boston Med Surg J.* **148**: 608–11.

33   Merz BJ *et al.* (1993) Implant metastasis of gallbladder carcinoma in situ in a cholecystectomy scar: a case report. *Surg.* **114**: 120–4.

34   Padilla RS, Jermillo M and Chapman W (1982) Cutaneous metastatic adenocarcinoma of gallbladder origin. *Arc Dermatol.* **118**: 515–17.

35   Rousselot R (1964) Tumeur ombilicale, metastase révélatrice d'un cancer vésiculaire. *Bull Soc Fr Derm Syph.* **71**: 670–2.

36   Hughes ES *et al.* (1983) Tumor wall recurrence in the abdominal wall scar after large bowel cancer surgery. *Dis Colon Rec.* **26**: 571–2.

37   Pool EH and Dunlop GR (1934) Cancer cells in the bloodstream. *Am J Surg.* **21**: 99–102.

38   Engell HC (1955) Cancer cells in the circulating blood. *Acta Chirurg Scand.* (Suppl.) **201**: 1–70.

39   Goligher JC, ed. (1984) *Surgery of the Anus, Rectum and Colon*, 5th edn. Baillière Tindall, London.

40   Engell HC (1959) Cancer cells in the blood. A five to nine year follow-up study. *Ann Surg.* **149**: 457.

41   Leather AJM *et al.* (1993) Detection and enumeration of circulating tumour cells in colorectal cancer. *Br J Surg.* **80**: 777–780.

42   Umpleby HC *et al.* (1984) Viability of exfoliated colorectal carcinoma cells. *Br J Surg.* **71**: 659–63.

43   Pomeranz AA and Garlock JH (1955) Postoperative recurrence of cancer of colon due to desquamated malignant cells. *JAMA.* **158**: 1434.

44   Quan SHQ (1959) Cul-de-sac smears for cancer cells. *Surg.* **43**: 258.

45   Moore GE *et al.* (1961) Assessment of the exfoliation of tumor cells into the body cavities. *Surg Gynec Obstet.* **112**: 469.

46   Juhl H *et al.* (1994) Immunocytological detection of micro-metastatic cells: comparative evaluation of findings in the peritoneal and pancreatic cancer patients. *Int J Cancer.* **57**: 330–5.

47   Schlimok G *et al.* (1990) Epithelial tumour cells in bone marrow of patients with colorectal cancer: detection, phenotypical characterisation and prognostic significance. *J Clin Oncol.* **8**: 831–7.

48   Lindemann F *et al.* (1992) Prognostic significance of micrometastatic tumour cells in bone marrow of colorectal cancer patients. *Lancet.* **340**: 685–9.

49   Rosenberg IL, Russell CW and Giles GR (1978) Cell viability studies on the exfoliated colonic cancer cell. *Br J Surg.* **65**: 188–90.

50   Fermor B *et al.* (1984) The proliferative and metastatic potential of exfoliated colorectal carcinoma cells. *J Nat Cancer Inst.* **74**: 1161–8.

51   Skipper D *et al.* (1987) Exfoliated cells and in vitro growth in colorectal cancer. *Br J Surg.* **74**: 1049–52.

52   Tanida O *et al.* (1982) Viability of intraperitoneal free cancer cells in patients with gastric cancer. *Acta Gytol.* **26**: 681–7.

53   Iitsuka Y *et al.* (1979) Intraperitoneal free cancer cells and their viability in gastric cancer. *Cancer.* **44**: 1476–80.

54   Sugarbaker V, Ketcham A and Cohen AM (1971) Studies of dormant tumor cells. *Cancer.* **28**: 545–52.

55   Fisher B, Fisher ER and Feduska N (1967) Trauma and the localization of tumor cells. *Cancer.* **20**: 23–30.

56 Davidson RB, Sams VR and Styles J (1990) Detection of occult nodal mestases in patients with colorectal carcinoma. *Cancer.* **65**: 967–70.

57 Philips RK *et al.* (1984) Local recurrence following 'curative' surgery for large bowel cancer: I. The overall picture. *Br J Surg.* **71**: 12–16.

58 Abulafi AM and Williams NS (1994) Local recurrence of colorectal cancer: the problem, mechanisms, management and adjuvant therapy. *Br J Surg.* **81**: 7–19.

59 Nicolson G (1988) Organ specificity of tumor metastasis: role of preferential adhesion, invasion and growth of malignant cells at specific secondary sites. *Cancer Metast Rev.* **7**: 143–88.

60 Poupon MF (1991) *La Dissémination Métastatique des Cellules Cancéreuses in Biologie des Cancers*, Ellipse, Paris. pp. 126–149.

61 Ryall C (1907) Cancer infection and cancer recurrence: a danger to avoid in cancer operations. *Lancet.* **ii**: 1311.

62 Killinback M, Wilson E and Hughes ESR (1965) Anal metastases from carcinoma of the rectum and colon. *Aust NZ J Surg.* 34–178.

63 Akyol AM *et al.* (1991) Anastomotic leaks in colorectal cancer surgery: a risk factor for recurrence? *Int J Colorectal Dis.* **6**: 179–83.

64 Zirngibl H, Husemann B and Hermanek P (1990) Intraoperative spillage of tumour cells in surgery for rectal cancer. *Dis Colon Rectum.* **33**: 613–14.

65 Patel Sc, Tovee EB and Langer B (1977) Twenty-five years experience with radical surgical treatment of carcinoma of the extraperitoneal rectum. *Surg.* **82**: 460–5.

66 Folkman J and Kalgsbrun M (1987) Angiogenic factors. *Science.* **235**: 442–7.

67 Paget S (1989) Distribution of secondary growths in cancer of the breast. *Lancet.* **ii**: 571–3.

68 Skipper D *et al.* (1989) Enhanced growth of tumour cells in healing colonic anastomoses and laparotomy wounds. *Int J Colorect Dis.* **4**: 172–7.

69 Editorial (1992) Colons and keyholes. *Lancet.* **340**: 824–5.

70 Wexner SD and Cohen SM. Personal communication.

71 O'Riordain M, Ross JA and Fearon KCH (1994) The inflammatory and metabolic response to open surgery and minimally invasive surgery. In: Brown S, Garden J (eds) *Principles and Practice of Surgical Laparoscopy.* W.B. Saunders, London. pp. 7–21.

72 Ramos J, Gupta S, Anthone G *et al.* Personal communication.

73   Beart RW (1994) Laparoscopic colectomy: status of the art. *Dis Colon Rect.* **37**: 47–9.

74   Fielding LP (1988) Surgeon-related variability in the outcome of cancer surgery. *J Clin Gastroenterol.* **10**: 130–2.

75   Turnbull RS *et al.* (1967). Cancer of the colon: the influence of the 'non-touch isolation' technique on survival rates: *Ann Surg.* **166**: 420–5.

76   Docherty JG *et al.* (1994) Local recurrence of colorectal cancer: the problem, mechanisms, management and adjuvant therapy. *B J Surg.* **81**: 1079–84.

77   Archer S and Gray B (1990) Intraperitoneal 5-fluoro-uracil infusion for treatment of both peritoneal and liver micrometastases. *Surg.* 1990: **108**: 502–7.

78   Philips EH *et al.* (1992) Laparoscopic colectomy. *Ann Surg.* 1992; **216**: 703–7.

79   Monson JRT *et al.* (1992) Prospective evaluation of laparoscopic-assisted colectomy in an unselected group of patients. *Lancet.* **340**: 831–3.

80   Falk PM *et al.* (1993) Laparoscopic colectomy: a critical appraisal. *Dis Colon Rect.* 1993; **36**: 28–34.

81   Eubanks S, Newman L, Lucas G (1993) Reduction of HIV transmission during laparoscopic procedures. *Surg Laparosc Endosc.* **3**: 2–5.

82   Moertel CG *et al.* (1990) Levamisole and fluoro-uracile for adjuvant therapy of resected colon carcinoma. *N Eng J Med.* **322**: 352–8.

83   Gerard A *et al.* (1988). Preoperative radiotherapy as adjuvant treatment in rectal cancer. Final results of a randomised study of the European Organisation for Research and Treatment of Cancer (EORTC). *Ann Surg.* **203**: 606–14.

84   American Society of Colon and Rectal Surgeons (1992). Policy statement. *Dis Colon Rect.* **35**: 5A.

85   SAGES (1991) Granting of privileges for laparoscopic general surgery. *Am J Surg.* **161**: 324–5.

15

Future trends in minimal access surgery: telepresence surgery and virtual reality

IRWIN B SIMON

Introduction

The concept of minimal access surgery was put under the surgical spotlight in 1989 with the advent of laparoscopic cholecystectomy[1]. This can be said to represent all the advantages and disadvantages of minimal access techniques. For the surgeon, high-tech devices for access and visualization bring their own problems. The charged coupled device (CCD) chip camera delivers only a two-dimensional image by way of the video monitor. Depth perception is sacrificed. Furthermore, the surgeon loses the ability to feel the patient's tissues manually; instead he must prod around with a limited array of laparoscopic instruments.

Robotics

Once again the medical world is turning to the scientific and engineering community to solve these problems, and telepresence surgery[2] may provide the solutions. First we must define a few terms[3]. *Robotics* is the science and art of performing, by means of an automatic apparatus or device, functions normally ascribed to human beings. *Teleoperation* is the extension of a person's manipulation capability to a remote location. Teleoperation refers to direct and continuous human control (one-to-one) of the remote manipulator. *Telerobotics* is a form of teleoperation in which a human operator acts as supervisor. The telerobot executes the task based on information received from the human operator plus its own artificial sensing and intelligence. With *telepresence*, information about the remote manipulator and task environment is communicated to the human operator in such a way that he feels as if he were physically present at the remote site.

Robotic technology is already being utilized in surgical procedures. Robo-Doc (Sacramento, California) is a robotic arm that follows computer guidance from a preoperative CT scan and can drill a femur with extreme precision, allowing the surgeon to press-fit a hip prosthesis. The Food and Drug Administration approved the first human trials, and the first human cases were reported on local and network news in November, 1992.

In the UK, similar technology has been utilized by Drs Timoney and Wickam. Their robotic surgery for transurethral resection of the prostate was the first totally robotic surgical procedure[4]. The limitation of this technology, however, is that the surgeon cannot impart his own knowledge and skills to the robot. This type of technologic assistance would fail in the thoracic cavity or the abdomen, where the organs are moving with respiration, where they move physiologically with peristalsis, and where the size and location of the target organ and/or tumor has great variability.

Telepresence remote surgery

The Green Telepresence Surgery System (SRI International, Menlo Park, California) is the prototype telepresence surgery system. It consists of an operating table where the telepresence remote surgery takes place and a surgical workstation from which the surgeon controls the procedure.

At the operating table, dual CCD cameras function with 'field sequential vision'. They go on and off faster than the human eye can discern: thus the image presented at the workstation is flicker-free. The operating surgeon wears simple polarizing glasses. The resulting image is perceived by the operating surgeon as a three-dimensional image.

The surgeon grasps simple hand controllers, and his motions are directly imparted through a computer interface to the teleoperator (robotic arm). The robotic arms are designed to impart a sensation of force feedback, via the computer interface, back to the hands of the operating surgeon. Weight and strength of pulling (as in tying an intracorporeal suture) are perceived by the surgeon at his workstation.

These motions are one-to-one in real time, with no discernible delay. The articulated arms allow multiple degrees of freedom and extreme precision of instrument control and placement. The result is a well integrated system that offers the surgeon the ability to operate deftly, as if he were actually present at the operative site.

The distance between the operative site and the surgeon's workstation is inconsequential. For obvious reasons, the first human applications will undoubtedly occur with the surgeon in the same room: but fiberoptic and satellite networking make extremely remote surgery a real possibility. A surgeon in a distant city or another part of the world may assist the local surgeon in an operative procedure. Time and cost savings may then offset the initial cost of bringing these technologies on line.

In the future, 3D imaging technologies (ultrasound, computed tomography, magnetic resonance imaging) may be blended into the surgeon's visual field.

Thus computer-assisted 'X-ray vision' can be anticipated as an offshoot of telepresence technology. The surgeon's ability to operate may be aided by superimposing these 3D images over the intraoperative image, enhancing the precision of the operation.

Virtual reality

The issue of surgical training has become more complex since the advent of minimal access surgery. How do we train young residents to perform operations on organs that they never actually see or feel? How do we train established surgeons in new techniques and the use of these new technologies?

The answer lies in the concepts of simulation. Military fighter pilots and commercial aviators do not fly multimillion dollar aircraft until they have 'flown' hundreds of hours in computer simulation. Virtual reality is a computer science in which virtual (artificial) worlds are created by computer-assisted design.

These 3D worlds can be quite realistic. An individual may become immersed in the virtual world by isolating his senses. This is usually achieved by wearing stereo video images, along with stereo audio input and some sort of joystick or DataGlove (VPL Research, Redwood City, California) device that allows the individual to interact (through the computer interface) with the artificial objects in the virtual world.

Current virtual reality technology does not yet provide truly realistic images, nor are the interactions effected in real time. These limitations are mainly those of the current generations of affordable computers. However, in the next five to 10 years we should see realism in computer simulation. This will undoubtedly involve a blend of computer-assisted design, computerized tomography, ultrasound, magnetic resonance imaging and digitized video from real operations.

The input device that allows interaction with a virtual reality surgical simulator must be realistic as well. The pilot trains in a simulator that looks just like the cockpit of his real aircraft. The surgeon will train at a computer workstation that looks and feels just like his real surgical workstation. The obvious solution is the marriage of telepresence and virtual reality.

The telepresence workstation may be utilized in a simulator mode. The image that the surgeon sees, and the tactile sensations he receives, must look and feel realistic. After demonstrating competence in multiple simulated patients and situations, the surgeon trainee may then be allowed to operate (with appropriate guidance) on real patients. Such simulators will allow training in both open and closed procedures. New procedures may be developed by surgeons with minimal need for animal experimentation prior to introduction in human protocols.

Future possibilities

Government and private sectors have seen the need for cost-effective advances in minimal access surgery as well as the need for surgical simulation. Today, the ability to limit blood exposure to the operating team is a significant rationale behind the possibilities of remote surgery. Remote operation decreases the possibility of transmission of infectious diseases, such as AIDS or hepatitis, to or from the patient.

As surgeons in all specialties continue to 'push the envelope' of minimal access surgery, we must find a time-effective and cost-effective way of performing these procedures. It is not acceptable to the patient, the surgeon, the government or third-party payee to convert a simple one-hour open operation to a difficult 12-hour minimal access procedures under general anesthesia. Telepresence offers one such approach.

Space exploration provides an exciting illustration of the need for telepresence surgery. It is not cost-effective to maintain a surgeon on call on the first space stations. However, when the first space station inhabitant develops appendicitis, a technician may prepare him for surgery, allowing the surgeon to perform the operation deftly from mission control via telepresence.

Brachytherapy (implantation of radioactive material directly into a malignant tumor) may be performed safely, with minimal exposure to operating room personnel, by precise surgery performed via telepresence. Cancer patients may also benefit from minimal access operations that might otherwise—without the aid of telepresence—have required open surgery.

Simulation for training must include the marriage of telepresence and virtual reality. Such virtual reality surgical simulators[5] appear to be on the near horizon as a cost-effective answer to some of the most important ethical issues that face the surgical world today.

Telepresence surgery and virtual reality for surgical simulation both arise from computer and communications technologies. These twin technologic advances have the potential to be the fundamental building blocks of the future of minimal access surgery.

References

1   Dubois F *et al.* (1990) Coelioscopic cholecystectomy. *Ann Surg.* **211**: 60–2.

2   Green PE *et al.* (1991) Telepresence: dexterous procedures in a virtual operating field. *Am Surg.* **57**: 192. (Abstract.)

3   Sheridan TB (1989) Telerobotics. *Automatica.* **25**: 487–507.

4   Timoney A *et al.* (1991) The use of robots in surgery. The development of a frame for prostatectomy. *J Endourol.* **5**: 165–8.

5   Satava RM (1993) Virtual reality surgical simulator; the first steps. *Surg Endosc.* **7**: 203–5.

Index

Since the major subject of this book is laparoscopic surgery, few entries are listed under this keyword. Readers are advised to seek more specific references.

abandonment of minimal access
    procedure 2
abdominal distension, contraindication to
    laparoscopy 7
abdominal evaluation, diagnostic
    laparoscopy 4–20
    see also diagnostic laparoscopy
abdominal lymph nodes *see entries*
    beginning lymph node
abdominal lymphomas *see* lymphoma,
    abdominal
abdominal wall
    lifting devices 177
    tumor implantation 27
acquired immune deficiency syndrome *see*
    AIDS
adhesions, relative contraindication to
    laparoscopy 7
adrenal adenoma 110
adrenalectomy 109–10
    bilateral 109
    indications 116
    surgical approaches 109
adrenalectomy, laparoscopic 110–17
    complication 115
    contraindications 110–11
    disadvantages 117
    flank *vs* anterior approach 116
    indications 110, 116
    left, procedure 112–13, 116
    open techniques *vs* 109–10

operative times 116–17
patient positioning 112, 114, 116
patient preparation 111
postoperative care 115
results 115–16
right, procedure 113–14, 117
technique 111–14
adrenal gland, medullary cysts 110
adrenal masses, resection 109–18
    see also adrenalectomy
adrenal tumors 110
adrenal vein, in laparoscopic
    adrenalectomy 113, 114
AIDS
    Kaposi's sarcoma in 70
    laparoscopic-directed biopsy in 8
    splenectomy in 75
aldosteronoma 110
American Cancer Society 21
American Society of Colo-Rectal Surgeons
    (ASCRS) 175
ampullary cancer 27
    diagnostic laparoscopy and biopsy 7–8
anesthesia
    laparoscopic adrenalectomy 111
    in laparoscopic staging 27
    thoracoscopy in solitary pulmonary
        nodules 137
angiogenesis, metastasis
    development 173, 175
angiomyolipoma

adrenal gland 110
splenic involvement 70
angiosarcoma, splenic 67
anterior resection, laparoscopic,
    metastases after 161
aortopulmonary window, thoracoscopic
    biopsy technique 141, 142
appendectomy, laparoscopic 90
ascites
    aspiration, sampling at laparoscopy 10
    intractable
        contraindication to laparoscopy 6
        control 17
        diagnostic laparoscopy in 14–17
ascitic leak 14
    avoidance 14, 17
atelectasis 82

Babcock forceps 59
barium enema 95
bile leak 28
biliary bypass
    laparoscopic 57–62
        indications 57, 62
        see also cholecyst-jejunostomy
    surgical 57–8
biliary-enteric anastomoses 26
biliary tree
    malignant obstruction 57
        see also common bile duct
    tumors, occult 27
biopsy
    radiographic-directed, laparoscopic
        biopsy *vs* 5
    in surgical staging of lymphomas 36–7
    transthoracic needle aspiration
        (TNAB) 135
    see also liver biopsy; lymph node
        biopsy
biopsy, laparoscopic 4, 11–14
    advantages 7–8
    core biopsy specimens 11–12, 14
    dissection of specimen 12, 15
    excisional 9, 13
        technique 13–14
    in high-risk patients 8
    incisional 9, 11
        lymph nodes 50
        technique 11–13
    indications 5–6
        metastases diagnosis 6
        staging 6, 7
    in pancreatic carcinoma 26

retroperitoneal 49–50
sample size 9
shave specimens 12, 15
techniques 11–14
thoracoscopic, of aortopulmonary
    window 141, 142
tissue removal methods 9
see also diagnostic laparoscopy; lymph
    node biopsy
bleeding, after laparoscopic splenectomy
    83
blood, tumor dissemination 169–70, 172
bone marrow biopsy, in non-Hodgkin's
    lymphoma 33
bowel preparation 95, 111
brachytherapy 28, 186
breast carcinoma 13, 160
bronchoscopy, in solitary pulmonary
    nodule 135
bulldog clamps, laparoscopic 154, 155

cannulae, laparoscopic biopsy 12
carbon dioxide
    aspiration, tumor dissemination
        prevention 176
    insufflation 5, 111
cardiopulmonary consequences,
    pneumoperitoneum 27
cardiopulmonary reserve, limited,
    laparoscopy contraindication 6
Castleman's tumor 68
cautery injury, complication in
    laparoscopy 18
celiac nodes, biopsy, in Hodgkin's
    disease 41, 42
cell cycle, tumor development and 172
certification of surgeons 2, 27
cervical mediastinal exploration (CME)
    140, 141
Chamberlain procedure 141
charged coupled device (CCD) chip
    camera 183
chemotherapy
    in Hodgkin's disease 71, 72
    intra-arterial 153
    intraperitoneal 176, 177
    port-site metastasis prevention 176,
        177
    regional, laparoscopic *see under*
        hepatic malignancy
cholecystectomy, laparoscopic
    complications 27, 28
    metastases after 27, 161

port-site metastasis 161, 167
in regional chemotherapy with
    laparoscopic approach 155
cholecyst-jejunostomy
    laparoscopic 58–62
        assessment before 59
        closure 61
        indications 58–9, 62
        patient selection/preparation 58–9
        port sites 60
        postoperative care 62
        techniques 59–61
    surgical 58
choledocho-jejunostomy with Roux-en-Y
    58, 59
coagulopathy
    diagnostic laparoscopy in 17
    laparoscopic staging and 27
    relative contraindication to
        laparoscopy 6
celiac nodes, biopsy, in Hodgkin's
    disease 41, 42
colectomy, laparoscopic *see* colorectal
    resection
collection bag *see* specimen bag
colon cancer *see* colorectal cancer
colonic lymphoma 33
colonoscopy 94
colorectal cancer 94
    fixation and bowel wall involvement
        95
    hepatic metastases, regional
        chemotherapy 153–6
    lymph node metastases 92–3
    port-site metastasis 94, 162, 163,
        167–8
        mechanism 175–6
    prognostic factors 95–6
    recurrence 94
    splenectomy in 74
    spread/dissemination 169–71
        malignant cells in colon 160,
            172–3
        malignant cells in peritoneum 160,
            170–1, 172
        routes 172–3
colorectal resection
    extent 91
    laparoscopic 90–108
        complications 96
        intracorporeal 95
        lymph node data 92–3, 96–7
        mortality 96

operative time 96, 97
port-site metastasis 94, 162, 163,
    167–8, 175–6
preoperative management 94–5
results 96–7, 98–106
technique 91, 94–7
training for 97
trial 90–1
tumor implantation and recurrence
    94
    laparoscopically-assisted 95, 97
    local tumor recurrence after 94
    lymph node numbers 92, 93, 96
    open techniques, local recurrence 94
    surgical standards 91–3
        ligation of blood supply 91–2, 97
        lymph node data reporting 92–3,
            97
        'no-touch' technique 91, 176
colosplenic attachments 77, 78
colostomy, laparoscopic 95
common bile duct, malignant obstruction
    57
    cholecyst-jejunostomy *see*
        cholecyst–jejunostomy
    diagnostic studies 58
    endoprostheses 57–8
computed tomography (CT)
    diagnostic laparoscopy comparison
        7–8
    lung cancer staging 140, 142
    lymph node evaluation 46, 47, 48
contamination of organs, prevention 16,
    176–7
contraindications, for minimal access
    surgery 2
core biopsy
    lymph nodes 50
    specimens 11–12, 14
core biopsy needle 11
Cotswolds Staging Classification 34, 35
credentialing of surgeons 2, 27
cryotherapy 28
cup biopsy forceps, lymph node biopsy
    50
Cushing's disease 110, 116
Cushing's syndrome 110
cytologic sampling, at laparoscopy 10–11

Data Glove 185
defatting technique, lymph node
    identification 92, 93, 97
diagnostic laparoscopy 4–20

in abdominal lymphomas 31
advantages *vs* disadvantages 7–8
complications 8, 18
computed tomography comparison
    7–8
contraindications 6–7, 17
    absolute 7
    relative 6–7
future prospects 18
history 4–5
indications 5–6
mortality risk 27
samples obtained by 9
in special situations 14–17
    coagulopathy 17
    intractable ascites 14–17
staging of disease *see* laparoscopic
    staging
techniques 9–14
    cytologic sampling 10–11
    histologic sampling 11–14
    see also biopsy
upper gastrointestinal tract cancer 22
visual inspection importance 10
see also biopsy, laparoscopic
drains, metastases after use 163, 169
duodenal bypass 61
duodenal-jejunal flexure (DJF) 59

effusions 159
electrocautery 17
endoprosthesis, in common bile duct
    obstruction 57–8
endoscopic pulmonary resection 139
endoscopic retrograde
    cholangiopancreatography (ERCP) 58
endoscopic ultrasound (EUS)
    colorectal cancer 94
    lymph node evaluation 46, 47
enteral feeding tubes, laparoscopic
    placement 119–33
    see also jejunostomy, laparoscopic
esophageal carcinoma
    evaluation and management 22–3
    laparoscopic enteral feeding tube
        placement 119
    laparoscopic staging 23
    laparoscopy advantages in 22
    resection 23
    survival and prognostic predictors 22
European Organization for Research and
    Treatment of Cancer 72, 176
Ewing's sarcoma, laparoscopic biopsy 5

fiberoptics 5
fibrin, tumor cells binding to 164
fibrous histiocytoma, splenic involvement
    70
'field sequential vision' 184
fine needle aspiration/biopsy
    pancreatic carcinoma 26
    parietal metastases after 169
    sampling at laparoscopy 10–11
fluid aspiration, sampling at laparoscopy
    10
fluoroscopic guidance, enteral feeding tube
    placement 119
Fowler's position 114
future trends, in minimal access surgery
    183–6

gallbladder
    carcinoma, implantation during
        laparoscopy 27–8
    laparoscopic assessment before
        cholecyst-jejunostomy 59
gastrectomy
    partial, laparoscopic, metastases after
        161
    port-site metastasis after 161, 168
    radical, splenectomy with 74
gastric bypass, laparoscopic 57–62
    indications 57
gastric carcinoma
    dissemination 171
    incidence 21, 24
    laparoscopic enteral feeding tube
        placement 119
    laparoscopic lymph node dissection 25
    laparoscopic staging 24–5
    management 24–5
    splenectomy in 74
gastric lymph nodes, laparoscopic
    evaluation 48–9
gastric lymphoma 34
gastrointestinal tract
    cancer
        incidence and death rates 21
        spread, routes 172–3
        see also colorectal cancer; gastric
            carcinoma
    laparoscopic staging 21–30
    non-Hodgkin's lymphoma 33
gastro-jejunostomy 58
    procedure 61
gastrostomy, percutaneous endoscopic
    (PEG) 119

genetics, metastasis development 174
Green Telepresence Surgery System 184

hemangioma, splenic 66–7
hemangiosarcoma, splenic 67
hematoma
    after laparoscopic splenectomy 82
    splenic 66
hemolytic anaemia 73
hemorrhoidectomy, tumor implantation
    174
hemostasis, in lymph node biopsy 50
hairy-cell leukemia, splenectomy in 74
hamartoma, splenic 67–8
Hasson technique 24, 111, 113
hepatic artery catheterization,
    chemotherapy via 153–6
hepatic malignancy
    intra-arterial chemotherapy 153
    laparoscopic approach for regional
        chemotherapy 153–7
        case report 153–6
        further cases reports 156
        procedure 154–5
        results 156
    see also hepatocellular carcinoma
hepatic metastases
    diagnostic laparoscopy 5–6
    in pancreatic carcinoma 25
    regional chemotherapy 153–6
hepatocellular carcinoma
    laparoscopic biopsy and port-site
        metastasis 168
    see also hepatic malignancy
hernias 82
histologic sampling, at laparoscopy
    11–14
    see also biopsy, laparoscopic
Hodgkin's disease 34–6
    classification and staging system 5, 34
    course of 34
    diagnosis and evaluation 34
    extranodal disease 34
    laparoscopic staging 32, 52–4, 72
        see also under lymphoma,
            abdominal
    splenic involvement 68
    staging laparotomy 31–2, 35–6, 72
    treatment
        chemotherapy 71, 72
        historical aspects 71
        splenectomy see splenectomy
    stage I/IIA 35

stage IIB 36
stages III/IV 36, 72
surgery role 71–3
hypersplenism 73
    splenectomy in 75

iliac nodes, biopsy, in Hodgkin's disease
    41
immunization, before splenectomy 76
immunology, metastasis development 174
incisions, VATS lobectomy 145
indications, for minimal access surgery 1
infections, after laparoscopic
    splenectomy 82, 83
inguinal nodes, biopsy, in Hodgkin's
    disease 41
instruments
    laparoscopic splenectomy 78–9
    lymph node biopsy 50–1
insufflation 5, 111
    history 5
interferon-alpha 74
intestinal lumen, exfoliated cells in and
    tumor spread 170, 172–3
    viability of 171
intra-abdominal pressure 3
intra-abdominal resections 3
    see also colorectal resection
intraluminal spread of tumors 170, 172–3
intraperitoneal adhesions 7
intraperitoneal dissemination of tumors
    170–1, 172

jejunostomy, percutaneous endoscopic
    119
jejunostomy, laparoscopic 119
    disadvantages 131
    extracorporeal vs intracorporeal
        method 131
        intracorporeal suturing
            disadvantage 131
    indications 119
    methods 120–30
        exteriorization method 120–3
        intracorporeal suturing method
            122, 123–30
    operative time 130
    patient selection 119–20
    postoperative recovery 121, 123
    results 130
jejunum, proximal, identification 121

Kaposi's sarcoma, splenic involvement 70

Keith needle 123, 124, 125

laparoscopic biopsy *see* biopsy,
    laparoscopic
laparoscopic evaluation, lymph nodes
    48–9
    see also under lymphoma, abdominal
laparoscopic staging 6, 7, 21–44
    abdominal lymphomas *see* lymphoma
    complications 27–8
    contraindications 27
    future directions 28
    gastric carcinoma 24–5
    mortality risk 27
    esophageal carcinoma 23
    pancreatic carcinoma 25–6
    upper gastrointestinal tract 21–30
    *see also specific organs/anatomical
        regions*
laparoscopic ultrasound, in colorectal
    resections 95
laparoscopy
    atlas of 48
    diagnostic *see* diagnostic laparoscopy
    history 4–5
    origin of term 4
    see also individual procedures
laparotomy
    Hodgkin's disease staging 31–2, 35–6,
        72
    laparoscopic biopsy comparison 5
    in lymphomas 31, 35–6, 72, 73
laser
    injury, complication in laparoscopy 18
    lung resection 139
leukemia, splenectomy in 73
lipoma, splenic involvement 70
liver
    disease, advantage of
        laparoscopic-directed biopsy 8
    metastases *see* hepatic metastases
    in non-Hodgkin's lymphoma 33
liver biopsy
    laparoscopic, in Hodgkin's disease
        38–9, 40
    percutaneous, in Hodgkin's disease 32
lobectomy, thoracoscopic 139
lung cancer
    resection *see* lung resection
    staging 140–7
        cervical mediastinal exploration
            (CME) 140, 141
        intraoperative 142, 143

        thoracoscopic 141, 142, 150
        treatment during thoracoscopy 135,
            143–4
        see also VATS lobectomy
    see also thoracoscopy
Lung Cancer Study Group 144
lung resection 143
    endoscopic 139
    laser 139
    thoracoscopic 135, 143–4
        nodules resection 137–9
    video-assisted lobectomy *see* VAT
        lobectomy
    wedge 143–4
lymphadenectomy, laparoscopic 51–2
    in colorectal cancer 92–3
    development of procedure 51
    extraperitoneal approach 51
    in gastric carcinoma 25
    in ovarian cancer 52
    'pelviscopie retroperitoneale
        panoramique' (PRPP) 51
    in prostate cancer 52, 53
    retroperitoneal approach 52
    transperitoneal approach 51
lymphangiography 45
    lymphoma staging 37
    technique 45, 46
lymphangiomas, splenic 67
lymphatic spread, of tumors 172
lymph node(s)
    in colorectal cancer, reporting of data
        92–3, 97
    identification, defatting technique 92,
        93, 97
lymph node biopsy 50–4
    development of procedures 50–1
    'incisional' 50
    instruments 50–1
    laparoscopic
        in Hodgkin's disease 41, 42
        in non-Hodgkin's lymphoma 33
    specimen management, in lymphomas
        37
    in surgical staging of lymphomas 37
    techniques 50–1
lymph node dissection *see*
    lymphadenectomy
lymph node evaluation 46–50
    in colorectal cancer 92–3
    future prospects 54
    historical aspects 45
    laparoscopic 48–9

in Hodgkin's disease 52
retroperitoneal, by laparoscopy 49–50
techniques (non-invasive) 46–8
lymph node excision 51
  in colorectal cancer 92–3
  see also lymphadenectomy
lymphoma, abdominal 31
  histiocytic, of spleen 69
  Hodgkin's *see* Hodgkin's disease
  laparoscopic staging 31–44, 37–43
    advantages 43
    Hodgkin's disease 38–43, 52–4, 72
    indications 37–8
    liver biopsy 38–9, 40
    lymph node biopsy 41, 42
    non-Hodgkin's lymphoma 33, 73
    operating room set-up 38
    results 42–3, 72
    splenectomy 39–41, 75, 80, 81
    techniques 38–42
    see also splenectomy
  non-Hodgkin's 32–4
    see also non-Hodgkin's lymphoma
  splenic involvement 68
  surgical staging 31–2, 36–7
    Hodgkin's disease 35–6, 72
    non-Hodgkin's lymphoma 33, 73
    post-operative and recovery 37
    procedure 36–7
  treatment 31
    surgery role 71–3

magnetic resonance imaging (MRI) 47–8
malignant fibrous histiocytoma 70
mediastinoscope 141
mediastinoscopy 141
melanoma, malignant, dormancy 160
mesenteric lymph nodes
  biopsy, in Hodgkin's disease 41
  resection, in colorectal cancer 93
mesothelioma, scrape specimens from 12
metastases
  after laparoscopy *see* port-site
    metastasis; tumor implantation
  definition 158
  development 172, 173–5
    biological factors in 174–5
    implantation *see* tumor
      implantation
    mechanisms 173–5
    vascular mechanism 173
  diagnosis, laparoscopic biopsy 6
  drains causing 163, 169

inoculation 159
  in open surgery 160–1, 168–9, 174
  'metastases following minimal access
    surgery' 162, 164
  see also port-site metastasis
metastatic potential, of tumors 169–71
micro-metastases 171
minimal access surgery
  abandonment of procedure, threshold
    2
  advantages 2
  contraindications 2
  duration/prolongation avoidance 2
  exposure needed 2
  future trends 183–6
  indications 1
  open procedures *vs* 1
  philosophy 1–3
multiple endocrine neoplasm (MEN-IIB)
  syndrome 110

National Cancer Institute (NCI) 32
natural killer (NK) cells 174, 175
Nd:YAG laser 139
needle jejunostomy tubes 131
needle placement, complication in
  laparoscopy 18
neoangiogenesis, metastasis development
  173, 175
nephrectomy, retroperitoneal
  laparoscopic 117
non-Hodgkin's lymphoma 32–4
  classification schemes 32
  colonic 33
  evaluation and investigations 32–3
  gastric 34
  liver involvement 34
  splenectomy in 73
  splenic involvement 68, 69
  staging 32, 73
  staging laparotomy 73
  surgeon's role in 33–4
  see also lymphoma, abdominal
no-touch technique 91, 176

oncological risks, of laparoscopic surgery
  166–82
  see also port-site metastasis
oophoropexy 37, 42
operating theatre, set-up in Hodgkin's
  disease staging 38
ovarian cancer
  laparoscopic lymphadenectomy 52

resection, port-site metastasis after 168
  splenectomy in 74
ovaries, shielding, in lymphomas 37, 42

palliative management, pancreatic cancer
  see pancreatic carcinoma
pancreas, laparoscopic approach 24
pancreatectomy 25
pancreatic carcinoma 21–30
  diagnostic laparoscopy and biopsy 7–8
  hepatic metastases in 25
  incidence and death rate 21, 57
  laparoscopic enteral feeding tube
    placement 119
  laparoscopic staging 25–6
    approach 25, 26
  occult tumor cell detection 25
  palliative management 25, 26, 57
    laparoscopic 58–62
    surgical 57–8
    see also cholecyst-jejunostomy
  port-site metastasis after laparoscopy
    168
  splenectomy in 74
pancytopenia 73
para-aortic nodes, laparoscopic
  lymphadenectomy 52
parietal metastases 168–9
patient positioning
  cardiopulmonary complication 27
  diagnostic laparoscopy 8
  laparoscopic adrenalectomy 112, 114,
    116
  laparoscopic approach for regional
    chemotherapy 154
  laparoscopic enteral feeding tube
    placement 120, 121
  laparoscopic splenectomy 76
  laparoscopic staging 27
    in Hodgkin's disease 38
patient preparation, laparoscopic
  adrenalectomy 111
patient selection
  laparoscopic cholecyst-jejunostomy
    58–9
  laparoscopic jejunostomy 119–20
  VATS lobectomy 144
pelvic lymphadenoscopy 51
pelvic lymph nodes, laparoscopic
  lymphadenectomy 52, 53
pelvis, anatomy 53
percutaneous endoscopic gastrostomy
  (PEG) 119

percutaneous endoscopic jejunostomy
  119
percutaneous fine-needle aspiration, in
  pancreatic carcinoma 26
periampullary cancer 57
  see also ampullary cancer
periaortic nodes, biopsy, in Hodgkin's
  disease 41
peritoneal carcinomatosis, nodules in
  168, 169
peritoneal fluid
  aspiration, sampling at laparoscopy
    10, 11
  malignant cells in 160, 163
peritoneal washing, sampling at
  laparoscopy 10
peritoneoscopy, in Hodgkin's disease 32
peritoneovenous shunt 17
peritoneum, malignant cells in 160, 163
  tumor spread 170–1, 172
phaeochromocytomas 110, 111, 116
philosophy, of minimal access surgery
  1–3
photodynamic therapy 176
plasmacytoma, spleen 69
pleural effusions, malignant, thoracoscopy
  in 148, 149
pleurodesis, talc 148, 149
pneumonectomy, VATS 147
pneumoperitoneum
  cardiopulmonary consequences 27
  complication in laparoscopy 18
  in laparoscopic adrenalectomy 110
  in laparoscopic staging 27
  positive-pressure 17
  in splenectomy 76
  tumor dissemination mechanism 175
portal lymph nodes, biopsy, in Hodgkin's
  disease 41, 42
port placement
  intracorporeal suturing of Witzel
    jejunostomy tube 123
  jejunostomy 120, 121
  laparoscopic staging in Hodgkin's
    disease 38, 39
  see also trocar placement
port-site metastasis 158–65, 166–82
  appearance and size 168
  case reports 161–2, 166–8
    cholecystectomy 161, 167
    colorectal cancer 162, 163, 167–8,
      175–6
  characteristics 168

explanation for 162–3, 164
interval after laparoscopy before
    detection 163
mechanisms 175–7
new terminology for 162
prevention 16, 176–7
see also tumor implantation
positron emission tomography (PET) 47,
    49
postoperative care
    laparoscopic adrenalectomy 115
    laparoscopic cholecyst-jejunostomy 62
    laparoscopic jejunostomy 121, 123
    laparoscopic splenectomy 82
    thoracoscopy 139–40
prostate cancer, laparoscopic
    lymphadenectomy 52, 53, 54
pseudocysts, splenic 64, 66
pulmonary arteries, in VATS lobectomy
    145
pulmonary complications, after
    laparoscopic splenectomy 82, 83
pulmonary lobectomy, video-assisted see
    videoassisted thoracic surgery
        (VATS)
pulmonary nodule, indeterminate solitary
    134
    management 134–40
        see also thoracoscopy
    numbers/incidence 135
pulmonary nodules, metastatic,
    thoracoscopy in 147–8

radiation, using laparoscopy 28
radioimmunologic-guided probes 18
radiolabeled antibody scanning, lymph
    node evaluation 47
radiotherapy, intraoperative 176
rectal cancer see colorectal cancer
rectum, laparoscopic anterior resection,
    metastases after 162
retroperitoneal biopsy 49–50
retroperitoneal mass, computed
    tomography-directed biopsy 48
retroperitoneoscopy 117
RoboDoc 184
robotics 183–4
Roux-en-Y choledocho-jejunostomy 58,
    59
Russell gastrostomy kit 125

sarcoma, splenic involvement 70
scrape specimens, obtaining 11, 12, 13

'second-look assessments', laparoscopy
    in 28
serosal wrap technique, jejunostomy
    feeding tube placement 121, 122
serous effusions 159
shave biopsy 12
space exploration, telepresence surgery
    186
specimen
    in laparoscopic splenectomy 39–41
    removal
        port-site metastasis prevention 176
        tumor dissemination mechanism
            175
        in VATS lobectomy 146
specimen bag 9, 13, 15, 16
    bowel bag in colorectal resection 94
    in laparoscopic splenectomy 39, 40,
        41, 80
    exteriorization 80, 81
spleen
    cystic lesions 64–6
    historical considerations 63–4
    laparoscopic evaluation and resection
        63–89
        see also splenectomy
    tumors see splenic tumors
splenectomy
    in colonic cancer 74
    in gastric cancer 74
    in hairy-cell leukemia 74
    historical considerations 63–4
    in Hodgkin's disease 32, 72–3, 73, 75
        laparoscopic 39–41, 75, 80, 81, 83
    in hypersplenism 73
    immunization before 76
    indications 64, 73
    infections after 64, 82, 83
    laparoscopic 75–6
        advantages 83
        complication rate 83
        complications 82–3
        in Hodgkin's disease 39–41, 75, 80,
            81, 83
        indications 75
        instruments 78–9
        open technique comparison 82, 83
        postoperative care 82
        procedure 39–41
        results 80–2
        specimen bag exteriorization
            71, 80
        specimen removal 39, 40, 41, 80

splenic artery embolization before
    76
        technique 76–80
    in leukemia 73
    mortality after 64
    in non-Hodgkin's lymphoma 73
    in ovarian cancer 74
    in pancreatic cancer 74
    in surgical staging of lymphomas 37
    techniques 75
        historical aspects 64
splenic artery embolization 39, 76, 77
    indications 76
splenic cysts 64–6, 65
    primary 64, 65
        keratinized 65
        parasitic and non-parasitic 65
    removal, historical considerations 64
    secondary 64, 66
splenic infarcts 75
splenic inferior/superior pole vessels,
    division 78, 79
splenic tumors 64–71
    categories 64
    clinical features 75
    lymphomas 68–9
    metastatic 68, 70
    non-lymphoid 70
    primary lymphoid 65, 68–9
        plasmacytoma 69
    primary non-lymphoid 65, 67–8
    pseudotumors 65
        see also splenic cysts
    secondary 68, 70
    splenectomy for 75
    vascular 65, 66–7
'splenoma' 67
splenomegaly 68, 75
splenophrenic attachments 78
sputum cytology 135
staging, diagnostic laparoscopy see
    laparoscopic staging
staplers
    in cholecyst-jejunostomy 60
    in laparoscopic splenectomy 79
    in VATS lobectomy 145, 146
subphrenic abscess 83
suture clips, tumor dissemination
    mechanism 175
suturing method, intracorporeal
    jejunostomy placement 122, 123–30,
    132

talc pleurodesis 148, 149
teleoperation 183
telepresence remote surgery 183, 184–5
telepresence workstation 184, 185
telerobotics 183
thoracoscopy 132
    advantages 148, 150
    evaluation and resection by 134–52
    explorative, in VATS lobectomy 145
    in indeterminate solitary pulmonary
        nodule 134–40
        advantage 135
        diagnosis 135, 136
        nodule resection 135, 137–9
        postoperative care 139–40
        preoperative needle localization
            135, 136, 137
        technique 137–40
    indications 135, 147, 148
    lung cancer staging 140, 141, 150
        intraoperative 142, 143
        left-sided cancer 141
    lung cancer treatment 135, 143–4, 159
        wedge resection 143–4
        see also VATS lobectomy
    in malignant pleural effusions 148,
        149, 150
    in metastatic pulmonary disease
        147–8, 150
    pneumonectomy 147
    wedge resection of lung 135, 143–4
thoracotomy, videoassisted 147
thromboembolic complications, after
    laparoscopic splenectomy 83
TNM system, esophageal carcinoma
    staging 23
touch preparations, sampling at
    laparoscopy 10, 11
training 2, 27
    colorectal resection 97
    telepresence and virtual reality 28, 186
transcelomic spread, of tumors 159
transthoracic needle aspiration biopsy
    (TNAB) 135
trauma
    laparoscopic enteral feeding tube
        placement 119
    metastasis development 174
    secondary (pseudo) cysts of spleen 66
Treitz, ligament of 121
trocar placement
    complication in laparoscopy 18

hepatic artery access for
  chemotherapy 154
laparoscopic adrenalectomy 112, 113
laparoscopic splenectomy 76
retroperitoneal inspection in
  esophageal carcinoma 23
thoracoscopy, in solitary pulmonary
  nodules 137
see also port placement
tuberculosis, peritoneal 10
tumoricidal agents 176, 177
tumor
  development 171–2
    metastases *see* metastases
    micro-metastases 171
  dormancy 160, 171–2
  invasion, pathogenesis 159
  removal *see* specimen removal
  spread 158–61, 169–71
    blood stream 169–70, 172
    digestive cancers 172–3
    direct 172
    intraluminal 170, 172–3
    intraperitoneal 160, 163, 170–1,
      172
    by laparoscopy *see* port-site
      metastasis
    steps in 159
    surgical
      transplantation/inoculation
      160–1, 168–9, 174
    transcelomic 159
    viability of cells 171
    see also tumor implantation
tumor cells, disseminated, viability 171
tumor implantation 18, 27–8, 159–60
  abdominal wall 27, 162
  case reports 161–2
  in colorectal resection 94, 162, 163
  evaluation of mechanism 162–3, 164
  in laparoscopic surgery *see* port-site
    metastasis
  mechanism 169, 173–4
  in open surgery 160–1, 168–9, 174
  see also port-site metastasis

ultrasonography

laparoscopic 6, 59
  lymph node evaluation 46–7
upper gastrointestinal tract *see*
  gastrointestinal tract

vascular mechanism, metastasis
  development 173
vascular tumors, of spleen 65, 66–7
VATS lobectomy 134, 139, 144–7, 150
  explorative thoracoscopy in 145
  left lower lobes 144
  operative times 147
  patient selection 144
  results and absence of benefits 147
  technique 144–6
    dissection 145
    incisions 144
    specimen removal 146
  see also thoracoscopy
VATS pneumonectomy 147
VATS Registry 139
vena cava, in laparoscopic adrenalectomy
  114, 117
venous dissemination, of tumors 172
'ventroscopy' 4
Verres needle
  ascitic leak prevention 14, 17
  in laparoscopic adrenalectomy 111
  in retroperitoneal laparoscopic
    nephrectomy 117
video-assisted thoracic surgery (VATS)
  132
  see also thoracoscopy; VATS
    lobectomy
video-assisted thoracotomy 147
video mediastinoscopy 141
videotaping 2–3
virtual reality 185

Witzel jejunostomy tube 122, 123, 131
  intracorporeal placement method 122,
    123–30
    results 130
  laparoscopic-assisted exteriorization
    method 120–3
    results 130, 131
  see also jejunostomy, laparoscopic